The Physician and Managed Care

by David E. Vogel

The Physician and Managed Care
by David E. Vogel

©1993 David E. Vogel
All Rights Reserved by the American Medical Association, 1993

ISBN 0-89970-570-7

Additional copies may be purchased from:
Order Department OP637393
American Medical Association
PO Box 109050
Chicago, IL 60610
Call 800 621-8335 for VISA, MasterCard,
American Express, or Optima orders.

DBA:93-526:5M:8/93

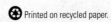 Printed on recycled paper.

Table of Contents

Acknowledgements

This book is the result of the support and assistance of several individuals. Sharyn Bills lent her highly-developed editing skills to the rewrite of the original manuscript. Ed Hirshfeld and Denise Andresen of the AMA staff contributed constructive comments and suggestions about how to make the work more helpful to physicians. Marietta Leis gave substantial time and energy to expediting the logistics and supporting the entire effort.

To each of these individuals, I extend my sincere appreciation for their help and expertise.

David E. Vogel
Corrales, New Mexico

Preface

Traditionally, the vast majority of physicians have practiced as solo practitioners or in small groups, and they have delivered services to patients on a fee-for-service basis. This method of practice allows individual physicians a tremendous amount of autonomy in their clinical and economic decision making. Reliance on the clinical and economic judgment of individual physicians has made American medicine the highest quality health care in the world.

In recent years, this system of delivering physician services has been challenged. The increasing cost of medical care and the large number of Americans who do not have assured access to health care services have caused alternative ways of delivering health care services to emerge. In this era of transition and experimentation, the American Medical Association (AMA) has stressed that traditional methods of delivering health care are the foundation of American medicine, that they continue to have value, and that they should not be abruptly dismantled in favor of new, unproven methods. The AMA believes that alternative methods of delivering care should be tested and made available, but that patients and physicians should have choices. The free market should determine the kind of systems and health plans that will be used based on the decisions made by patients and physicians.

Managed care is a nontraditional method of delivering health care that has become increasingly prevalent in recent years. Indeed, in a few markets in the United States, managed care has become the dominant method of financing and providing medical care. Projections are that the percentage of patients accounted for by managed care will continue to grow. As a result, many members of the AMA have asked for information about how managed care plans are organized and operated, how physicians can successfully practice in managed care plans, how physicians can organize their own networks to contract with managed care plans, and how physicians can form their own managed care organizations.

This book, *The Physician and Managed Care,* by David Vogel, is meant to provide the information that members are seeking. The book is an excellent introduction to the subject of managed care. It covers basic information about how managed care plans operate, organizational structures for physicians who wish to contract with managed care plans, and what is necessary to adapt a medical practice to managed care. The book is intended for physicians who know little about managed care and want to start learning. However, the book is comprehensive enough that physicians who are familiar with managed care will find that it can help fill gaps in their knowledge.

Physicians will have different reactions to the material in this publication. Some will find the information useful and stimulating. Others may feel differently, as they find it philosophically difficult to accept managed care as a part of the health care delivery system. However, the purpose of this book is to provide objective information about managed care for physicians who need it, not to promote managed care or any other delivery system. Further, the AMA believes that physicians are more likely to preserve their traditional autonomy in clinical and economic decision making if they understand managed care and how to practice successfully in a managed care environment. Physicians can and should serve as the focal point for clinical and economic decision-making in a managed care plan, and can do so if they have the knowledge and informational tools necessary.

This book is not an endorsement of managed care by the AMA and it does not enunciate AMA managed care policy. AMA policy about managed care is set forth in another publication in the Medicine in Transition series, entitled *Principles of Managed Care.* The *1993 Policy Compendium* of the American Medical Association also sets forth AMA managed care policy at pages 241-245.

On behalf of the American Medical Association, I hope that you will find the information in *The Physician and Managed Care* useful to you.

James S. Todd, M.D.

Introduction

At least 70 percent of the entire US population will be enrolled in some type of managed care program by the year 2000, most experts predict. By the end of this decade, the managed care industry will be serving a comprehensive spectrum of the US population, including those covered by commercially-insured managed care products, Medicare and Medicaid beneficiaries, and, if Congress passes guaranteed-access legislation, the medically-underserved. Although some geographically isolated areas of the country may remain untouched by this trend, it is expected that the vast majority of those living in the US will be participants in some managed care arrangement before the century ends. Few physicians will be immune from the effects of this trend.

Managed care is part of a broader effort to affect certain trends that are causing increasing distress to the US health care system. The increase in the percentage of Gross National Product spent on health care from 6 percent in 1965 to 14.4 percent in 1992 is but one of the major concerns that have resulted in many proposals for health care reform that currently are being considered at both the state and national level. The growing number of uninsured Americans is another.

How to resolve these cost and access issues are only two of the difficult questions facing our health care system. The problems are many; the solution or solutions therefore will have to be comprehensive rather than piecemeal. Managed care is only one of the solutions currently being proposed, and physicians themselves can resolve only some of the problems. However, each component of the health care system does have the potential to contribute something to the total solution. Physicians, hospitals, and other providers, consumers, employers, unions, health insurance companies, and managed care organizations all hold pieces that are essential to successfully putting together the puzzle of health care reform.

The solutions, when they come, undoubtedly will require significant change on the part of all those players, and it is not difficult to understand why the prospect of change causes so much anxiety. Nonetheless, many physicians are anxious to act now so that they may exert influence over the changes that are most likely to affect them. To prepare for and manage change, however, they need information. They need to recognize that they do have options. They need to know what those options are and how to exercise them effectively. It is the purpose of this book to help physicians achieve that understanding.

The health care industry in general, and the managed care component in particular, are being mandated by *society* — not by some arbitrary political agenda — to respond to the demand for better value and greater access. That is a fact that observers too often fail to recognize. There are no simple solutions to these complex social and economic issues, nor is managed care either a panacea or the only approach that has merit.

However, there are aspects of managed care that have the potential to provide some of the solutions to this country's current health care dilemma. The information presented in the following chapters can help physicians learn how to participate in managed care in a constructive and professionally rewarding way. The patient must always remain the primary focus of any discussion about health care access, quality, and cost, and physicians must remain the patient's advocate at all times.

Given market forces and legislative trends, continued and perhaps accelerated growth in managed care is a virtual certainty. While that fact may seem threatening to many, it is possible for physicians not only to cope with the new environment, but to thrive in it. It is the intent of this book to provide the informational tools that will make intelligent decision-making possible for the physician interested in constructively anticipating change.

Managed care is a subject that is open to many different points of view. Every effort has been made to present the information contained herein as objectively as possible, based on the author's almost 30 years of work in health care as a clinician, manager, and consultant. During his career, the author has worked with thousands of physicians to assist them in trying to cope with change, and his primary interest remains helping physicians learn to thrive within the context of change. It is the author's hope that the insights and perspectives gained from this experience will help the reader meet the challenges of the 90s.

One further point warrants emphasis. Physicians frequently ask how they can organize to deal with managed care. The best way to answer that question is to ask, in turn, *why* physicians may want or need to organize. All too often physicians' initial reaction to the perceived "threat" of managed care is to organize for the purpose of preserving the status quo, rather than for the purpose of maximizing the value of health care services provided. As we will see in the pages that follow, dozens of provider-sponsored managed care organizations failed during the 1970s and 1980s precisely for that reason. That fact suggests the wisdom of maximizing one's options rather than limiting them. It also emphasizes the importance of physicians clearly identifying their objectives *before* they organize so they can determine *if* organizing will help them meet their objectives, and then *what type* of entity might serve them best. It is hoped that the information provided in this book will support the physician in this kind of constructive decision-making.

Chapter 1:

The Vehicles of Managed Care

Managed care is a term that has come into common usage only during the past few years. Referring to a still evolving concept, its definition is by no means as yet commonly agreed upon. Indeed, to some extent, attempting to define the term reminds one of the fable of the blind men's description of an elephant — each individual's definition seems to depend upon which part of the beast he happened to encounter.

The Physician and Managed Care

Many definitions refer to managed care as the process of managing costs. For example, the National Association of Children's Hospitals has defined managed care as:

An attempt to contain health care costs by controlling how and where patients obtain health care services. Any health insurance or health financing control mechanism or financial inducement intended to direct or restrict the patient's choice of provider or the patient/physician's choice of treatment modality.

Physicians who have working knowledge of and experience in managed care may argue that truly effective managed care focuses on managing care rather than managing cost. Thus, for the purposes of this publication we prefer to define managed care as:

A means of providing health care services within a defined network of health care providers who are given the responsibility to manage and provide high quality, cost-effective health care to a defined population.

The term "managed care organization" (MCO) will be used throughout this document and is intended to generically include any of the managed care acronyms (HMO, CMP, IPA, POS, PPO, EPO, DPO, PHO). The term "provider" will be used to refer generically to individuals and organizations involved in providing care to patients (eg, physicians, hospitals, pharmacies, home health agencies, etc).

The Objectives of Managed Care

From a physician's perspective, it is essential to conceptually redefine managed care from this external definition:

Something that someone from the outside does to me.

to this more internalized concept:

A process that involves managing patients, referrals, admissions, discharges, ancillary services, resources, and outcomes.

This conceptual redefinition places the primary responsibility for clinical decision-making exactly where it belongs: with the physician.

To take this redefinition one step further, it should be recognized that care is almost always best managed at the point of the doctor-patient interface. This is where the clinical decision-making process needs to be supported by the MCO.

Unfortunately, most of the effort and attention of MCOs and physicians in the past has been committed to contractual matters, practice management matters, and other non-clinical issues. In fact, these non-clinical issues represent only a small part — perhaps no more than 15 percent — of what managed care is all about. To be successful, most of the efforts of a managed care organization must be focused on supporting the physician clinical decision-making process. Similarly, the primary focus of physicians in successful MCOs must be on the doctor-patient interface and the clinical processes that occur there.

By redefining managed care in this fashion, physicians can begin to take charge of the clinical elements of managed care while moving away from the former external "managed access" approach. If physicians do not manage care by managing patients, resources, and outcomes, the only options left for MCOs, insurance companies, and government is to artificially control cost and utilization by controlling access, discounting fees, and implementing price controls. These options are clearly undesirable for a whole host of reasons, including the fact that they impose administrative interventions upon the doctor-patient relationship.

If physicians are to be effective in leading health care reform and redefining managed care, they must become knowledgeable about the basic principles of managed care and the environment, or "market," in which managed care operates. To begin, physicians must understand the three primary objectives of managed care, which are (1) to maximize quality, (2) to maximize patient service, and (3) to minimize total cost per person per year.

When physicians and MCOs have accomplished all three of these objectives, they have maximized the *value* of the health care service they are providing to their patients and members. When value has been maximized, physicians and MCOs are producing what the health care market is demanding. It is becoming increasingly apparent that providers and MCOs that are market-driven and value-based in their provision of care will have the greatest likelihood of being rewarded with a steady flow of patients.

Historically, managed care organizations have focused on reducing the number of hospital days utilized per 1,000 population. They do so through a variety of approaches, among them, preadmission testing, concurrent utilization review, discharge planning, retrospective utilization review, second surgical opinion, same day surgery, home care, and case management. Such techniques have contributed to a continued steady decline in hospital days utilized per 1,000 population throughout the country. This trend is expected to continue throughout the 1990s.

> Although nonhospital, or ambulatory, services have not yet been as carefully managed by managed care organizations, they are expected to be a significant target in the current decade.

Although nonhospital, or ambulatory, services have not yet been as carefully managed by managed care organizations, they are expected to be a significant target in the current decade. Ambulatory services management techniques most typically used by MCOs include case management, drug formularies, practice management support systems, and referral authorizations for subspecialty, ancillary, and other non-primary care services.

MCOs may also attempt to achieve their objectives through the use of defined provider networks; benefits design, such as coverage limitations and expansions; cost sharing through copayments, coinsurance, and deductibles; provider incentive/risk-sharing systems; quality management systems; and management information systems.

An important distinction among the various definitions and "perspectives" of managed care lies in the focus and *intention* — the basic objectives — behind the MCO and its providers, the intention and focus of the major purchasers (employers, federal and state government), and how these intentions get translated into MCO organization structures, quality and utilization management systems design and operation, provider incentive system design, and a host of other "infrastructure" factors that significantly influence which perspective or definition actually is being operationalized within any given MCO. It is therefore important for the physician comparing or evaluating an MCO to objectively determine which perspective prevails.

Another important issue to clarify is who is actually "managing" the care: the MCO or the primary care physicians and the subspecialists to whom they refer? A primary function of the MCO is to provide support and an infrastructure that provides physicians with the tools that enable them to better manage care. Sometimes this occurs; sometimes it does not. The managed care industry is still developing, and the state of the art is such that some of these "tools" are still under development.

One factor that is critical to the success of MCOs is the quality of physicians they recruit. Lacking a strong physician base, no MCO can achieve its quality and cost objectives. At the same time, it is important to emphasize that no physician can manage care effectively without substantial support from the MCO. The kinds of supports that the MCO must provide are discussed in detail in Chapter 3. In reviewing them, it is important to keep in mind that these functions *must* be oriented toward assisting and supporting providers, and most importantly the physician providers, in managing care. Successful managed care requires interdependence between the MCO and its physicians. If this relationship does not facilitate a true "win/win" partnership, neither the physician nor the MCO can succeed at managed care.

> It is important to understand the distinction between managed care products and managed care delivery systems.

Defining what a specific managed care organization is and how it operates is an even more complicated task than arriving at a generic definition for the term managed care. In the process of their rapid evolution, literally dozens of different forms of these organizations have emerged, each with its own designation and acronym, its own underlying philosophy and method of operation. To further complicate the matter, variations may exist from organization to organization within each general category. While the following discussion will attempt to delineate distinctions among the various types of MCOs, it is important to be aware that, in this rapidly evolving field, distinctions are blurring.

To understand the world of managed care, it is also important to understand the distinction between managed care products — the various packages of services that are available to the purchaser — and managed delivery system models — the way in which providers are organized within and relate to an MCO.

HMOs, CMPs, PPOs, POSs, PPAs, EPOs, and DPOs are among the acronyms most commonly heard when the discussion turns to managed care. Let's examine what each signifies.

Managed Care Products

A managed care product is a package of insurance benefits that is combined with a specific network of doctors, hospitals, and other providers who are organized within certain kinds of health care delivery system models. For example:

Health Maintenance Organizations (HMOs)

Health Maintenance Organizations are responsible for both financing and providing an agreed-upon set of comprehensive health maintenance and treatment services to a specifically defined and voluntarily enrolled population for a prepaid, fixed sum. Thus, an HMO serves as both an insurer and a provider (or an arranger) of health care services. In contrast to traditional indemnity health insurance, which simply reimburses covered individuals or those who provide health care services to them, the close relationship between insuring and providing services requires HMOs and their providers to carefully monitor and manage both the quantity and quality of care.

HMOs are typically separated into five types — the staff model, the group practice model, the Individual Practice Association model, the direct contract model, and the network model. The significance of those categories will be discussed in the following section on delivery system models. For the moment, it is sufficient to note that, like so many other distinctions in managed care, the lines between these categories now appear to be blurring.

Competitive Medical Plans (CMPs)

Competitive Medical Plans are a type of managed care product created under 1982 federal legislation designed to facilitate the enrollment of Medicare beneficiaries in managed care plans. Organized and financed much like HMOs, but subject to fewer regulatory restrictions, CMPs did not experience much enrollment growth in their early years. However, as the federal government continues to seek more successful means of controlling the cost and quality of health care services provided to the elderly, it is likely that the managed care industry will become much more aggressive in the enrollment of Medicare beneficiaries.

Preferred Provider Organizations (PPOs)

Unlike HMOs, which are discrete, licensed insurance products, Preferred Provider Organizations represent arrangements between groups of physicians, hospitals, and other providers, and either a health insurance carrier, a third-party administrator, or a self-insured employer. These "preferred providers," as those selected providers are known, enter into a contract with the PPO, which can be an insurance company, a Blue Cross/Blue Shield plan, a third-party administrator (TPA), a large employer, an HMO, or an organization of doctors (and sometimes hospitals) that has been created specifically for this purpose. Under the contract, the providers agree to abide by certain rules, regulations, and procedures, such as utilization review and pre-certification, as well as to certain reimbursement arrangements, in exchange for an anticipated increased volume of patients. To complete the arrangement, PPO beneficiaries are offered financial incentives such as lower coinsurance payments and deductibles to seek care through the preferred providers. Unlike members of HMOs, these beneficiaries retain the option of seeking care from either the preferred providers or providers of their choice, if they are willing to pay the extra charges.

Typically, PPOs reimburse physicians at discounted fee-for-service rates, a primary means of attempting to reduce the cost of care to purchasers. However, the arrangement provides little incentive to physicians to manage care more effectively and may even have the opposite affect, as physicians attempt to make up revenues lost as a result of discounted fees. At the same time, unlike HMOs, which, in effect, limit beneficiaries to using their providers, PPOs offer consumers the option of whether or not to use a preferred provider. That difference further increases the difficulty of managing care.

In contrast to HMOs, PPOs do not assume the insurance risk for those consumers who participate in them. Thus, PPOs must be offered under the insurance license of an insurance company, a Blue Cross/Blue Shield plan, or an HMO, or under the auspices of a self-insured employer. Another important characteristic that distinguishes PPOs from HMOs relates to the way in which consumers who participate in them are described. Those who enter into an arrangement with an HMO are referred to as "members" who are said to "enroll" in the plan — that is, agree to receive practically all their health care from the HMO's providers. These consumers can therefore be said to be "locked in" to the HMO. In contrast, consumers who participate in a PPO agree only to receive care from the preferred providers if and when they choose to do so. Because they are not "locked in" to the PPO, they are said to be "eligible" to participate in it, rather than "enrolled" in it.

> Most HMOs are introducing POS products as a means of attracting greater market share than they can with the traditional "locked in" (to HMO providers) HMO product.

Point of Service Plans (POSs)

One of the fastest growing managed care products is the Point of Service (POS) plan. A POS product combines some of the features of an HMO with the provider selection flexibility of a PPO. Although there are many variations on the POS theme, in most cases members select a primary care physician who manages the patient's care. However, members have the ability to seek care from outside the POS network and have less coverage. Most HMOs are introducing POS products as a means of attracting greater market share than they can with the traditional "locked in" (to the HMO providers) HMO product.

Preferred Provider Arrangements (PPAs), et al.

Preferred Provider Arrangements (PPAs) involve contractual arrangements similar to those of Preferred Provider Organizations, except that the contracts are arranged for without the establishment of a separate organization to act as contracting agent. Under PPAs, an insurance entity contracts directly with individual physicians and other providers. Exclusive Provider Organizations (EPOs) and Designated Provider Organizations (DPOs) are variations on the same theme, except that they require their beneficiaries to use participating providers.

Hybrids of these products also exist, sometimes known as "opt-out," "swing,""leak," and "wrap" HMOs. These terms refer to variations on the basic HMO product design that are intended to permit beneficiaries greater flexibility in choosing providers. Indeed, many HMOs have also developed PPO-type products to diversify their product offerings.

Indemnity insurance carriers also have developed both HMOs and PPOs, as well as other managed care products. Thus, managed care organizations can be either discrete organizational entities or sponsored by an indemnity insurance company or Blue Cross/Blue Shield plan. Some have even been initiated by hospitals and/or physicians themselves.

Increasingly popular, too, is a method of packaging and marketing known as the "total replacement product." Typically, this kind of product consists of a combination of two or more managed care products with an indemnity product, which is offered by the sponsoring MCO in hopes of enrolling 100 percent of an employer group. These products are in contrast to the "dual choice" or "multiple choice" options some employers have offered, which permit employees to choose among managed care products sponsored by single-product MCOs, an option that creates complicated administrative problems for the employer.

Transition Products

Success in managed care requires an enormous amount of education on the part of all players — providers, consumers, and third parties alike. The development of transition products represents one managed care industry response to meeting that demand.

Recognizing the resistance of some consumers and providers to MCOs that limit flexibility, transition products involving relatively loosely-structured managed care may be introduced. Many PPOs may be transition products. Many PPO products that have been in existence for relatively long periods of time (given the newness of the whole idea of managed care) are gradually becoming more tightly structured as they attempt to have a greater impact on the cost and quality of care. The trend suggests that there may be greater readiness to accept more structured products by century's end. In fact, given the dynamic nature of the managed care industry, distinctions among terms such as HMO and PPO may soon come to be meaningless as the products they represent evolve in response to marketplace demands. This trend may well accelerate if certain health care reforms are enacted.

Meanwhile, some employers are demonstrating growing interest in directly contracting with providers for managed care services. Such arrangements are usually entered into by self-insured employers — that is, those that are large enough to underwrite their own health insurance. In such cases, an employer may use an insurance carrier to administer claims under a third-party administrator arrangement, but the employer continues to assume risk. Although it remains unclear whether this will become a significant trend, some physicians and hospitals have begun organizing themselves so that they will be able to directly contract with employers, should the marketplace demand such arrangements.

Direct contracting can, some believe, ultimately save employers certain "middle man" costs, while many providers expect direct contracting to mean higher levels of reimbursement for them. Too frequently overlooked is the fact that functions normally performed by third parties — functions such as claims, marketing, and delivery system management administration — still have to be performed, and that the costs of these functions will remain a factor, whatever the contractual arrangements. While it may be possible to eliminate some of the profit margin associated with insurance company costs, it should be noted that, except in unusual cases, insurance company profits historically have not been excessive.

Although some savings in administrative costs may be possible, it must be recognized that the essential services these administrative costs represent will not be eliminated with the elimination of a third party.

The realization that direct contracting would require employers or providers to develop insurance expertise and insurance operations capabilities may discourage some employers and providers. Employers may also be concerned about the liability implications of being closely associated with provider selection, as well as with employee and labor relations implications. Given those disincentives, the future of direct contracting remains uncertain.

Managed Fee-for-Service Plans

Sometimes included and sometimes excluded from discussions of managed care are what is known as "managed fee-for-service plans" — indemnity insurance, Blue Cross/Blue Shield, or employer self-insurance plans in which physicians are reimbursed on a fee-for-service basis. Such arrangements may incorporate mechanisms by which patients are directed toward specific providers, or through which services are bundled into units for the purpose of negotiating better prices with providers, or both. Managed fee-for-service plans also typically impose some form of control on the providers, such as preadmission certification or second surgical opinion requirements.

As of 1991, more than 80 percent of all employers incorporated some form of managed fee-for-service feature into their basic insurance plan. Although not now usually counted in compiling managed care statistics, it is likely that the numbers and impact of such arrangements will increase over time, and that they will eventually evolve into true managed care products.

Single Service Products

A single service managed care product is one that offers only one component of an MCO comprehensive benefits package. The most common examples are prescription drugs and mental health and dental services. Single-service MCOs specialize in their respective services only, and therefore frequently can offer an employer or a full-service MCO a significantly better value than the employer or MCO can produce on its own. The process of implementing these single-source products is frequently referred to as "unbundling," or "carving out," services.

Who's Buying What?

Managed care products operate within the general health insurance sector and therefore compete with indemnity health insurance plans, as well as with one another. It is important to note, however, that a particular managed care organization might offer a wide variety of managed care products in order to maximize its market share — that is, the percentage of a population that is captured by its managed care product line.

To better understand what is happening in managed care today, it is useful to arrange the various health insurance products on a spectrum (see Figure 1), ranging from those that are most tightly managed (HMOs) to those that are totally unstructured (standard indemnity insurance), together with the percentage of the total US population that currently participates in each.

> In the early 1970s, approximately 90 percent of the population of the US was covered by indemnity insurance products compared with only approximately 10 to 15 percent by 1991.

In the early 1970s, approximately 90 percent of the population of the US was covered by indemnity insurance products, including Blue Cross/Blue Shield plans, compared with only approximately 10 to 15 percent by 1991. The decline in indemnity insurance and the gradual but steady movement of health insurance products from left to right on this spectrum have been dramatic, and the trend is expected to continue through the 1990s. This is not to suggest that the entire population will eventually gravitate to HMOs. It does, however, suggest a continued movement toward more tightly managed products.

In reviewing this depiction of health insurance product trends, it is important to remember that, in contrast to the 1980s, when distinctions among the various types of managed care products and organizations were quite clear, those distinctions have now blurred considerably. For example, point-of-service (POS), or "open-ended," plans had become a popular HMO option by the early 1990s, permitting beneficiaries to opt out of the HMO's traditional closed panel of providers in the interest of making the traditional HMO product

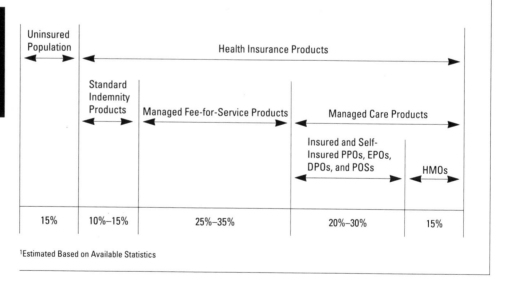

Figure 1
Current (1991) Health Insurance Product Line Spectrum and Market Share[1]

Uninsured Population

Health Insurance Products

Standard Indemnity Products

Managed Fee-for-Service Products

Managed Care Products

Insured and Self-Insured PPOs, EPOs, DPOs, and POSs

HMOs

| 15% | 10%–15% | 25%–35% | 20%–30% | 15% |

[1]Estimated Based on Available Statistics

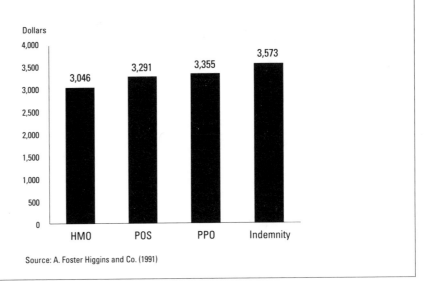

Figure 2
Average Health Care Costs Per Employee by Type of Product

Source: A. Foster Higgins and Co. (1991)

more attractive to potential members. Figure 2 illustrates the average cost per employee (including dependents) for employers by type of plan. A 1991 study conducted by the national benefits consulting firm A. Foster Higgins & Co. found a variation in cost of $500 per employee per year, based on the model.

Managed Delivery System Models

Behind every managed care product is a defined arrangement of physicians, hospitals, and other health care providers. What is known as the MCO's "health care delivery system," or "network," simply refers to the way in which these providers are organized.

Broadly speaking, there are five generally recognized delivery system models: the staff model, group practice model, network model, individual group practice model or Individual Practice Association (IPA), and direct contract model. These models are defined primarily by the relationship of participating physicians to the MCO. However, as is the case with managed care products, rapid evolution is the order of the day in managed care delivery system models as well.

Therefore, many variations on these basic models exist. In the wake of the constant quest of MCOs to capture larger and larger populations through diversification, hybridization is increasingly the norm. Numerous products can be offered through the same delivery system (although some models do permit greater product flexibility than others); thus, many MCO health care delivery system models are being continually broadened to include a wider selection of providers who can deliver a broader spectrum of products. For example, an MCO may utilize one tightly structured component of its total delivery system to service an HMO product, while utilizing a larger component to service a PPO product that it also offers.

How the health care delivery system is structured has a significant bearing on the ability of the MCO to manage care —that is, to have an influence over the use and cost of care. In turn, the degree of utilization and quality management capability structured into an MCO delivery system, as well as its size in terms of numbers of providers, determines its relative value and attractiveness to purchasers.

> How the health care delivery system is structured has a significant bearing on the ability of the MCO to manage care.

For example, the most tightly managed HMO model, the staff model HMO, theoretically is capable of maximum influence over the use and cost of care. However, because of the relatively small numbers of physicians who participate in a typical staff model HMO, and because enrollees are "locked in," or required to seek care only from participating providers if they wish the care to be paid for by the HMO, this model is likely to be less attractive to many potential enrollees. What the model gains in management capability, it may lose in marketability, unless the value of the MCO is perceived to be substantially higher. Because a physician's future may be tied to the future of an MCO he or she elects to participate in, understanding such variables is extremely important.

Staff and Group Practice Models

In the staff model MCO, individual physicians are employed directly by the managed care organization (see Figure 3), as compared to the group practice model, in which the MCO contracts with a physician group practice to provide services to its enrollees (Figure 4).

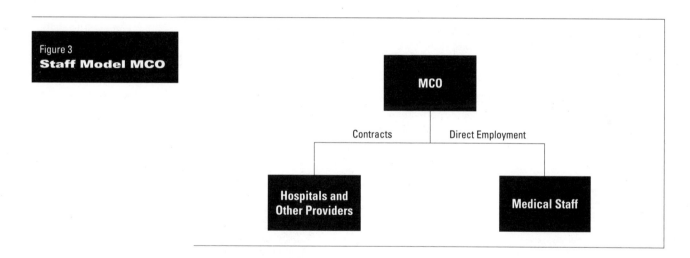

Figure 3
Staff Model MCO

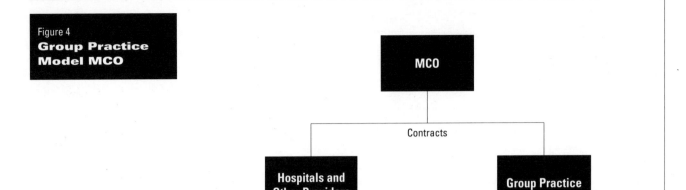

Figure 4
Group Practice Model MCO

Some group practices that participate in group practice model MCOs provide virtually 100 percent of their services to an HMO, as in the case of various Kaiser Foundation Health Plan HMOs operating in California, Colorado, the Pacific Northwest, and the mid-Atlantic states. Other group practices may have originally provided services on a fee-for-service basis, and subsequently entered the managed care arena. Among the latter group, the percentage of managed care patients typically gradually increases as local managed care market share increases. Staff and group practice MCOs have historically been referred to as "closed panel" models, while IPA-type MCOs have been called "open panel" models. This terminology has become obsolete as the distinctions between models have blurred.

The Network Model

Arrangements under the network model (Figure 5) are similar to those of the group practice model, except that instead of involving a single group practice, this model functions through a network of group practices, all contracting with the MCO. The group practices within the network may provide all of their services to one MCO, or they may be fee-for-service groups that provide only some of their services to one or more MCO.

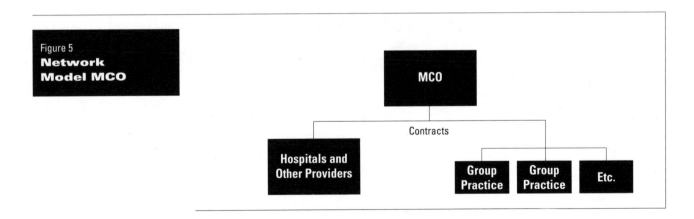

Figure 5
Network Model MCO

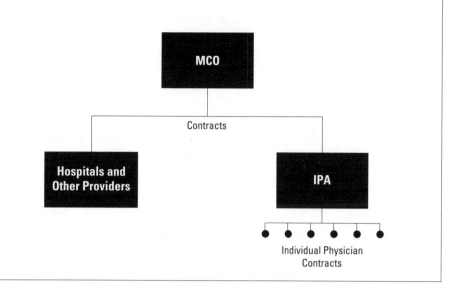

Figure 6
IPA-Type Model MCO

MCO

Contracts

Hospitals and Other Providers

IPA

Individual Physician Contracts

Variations on the network model include primary care group practice networks, which work primarily through primary care groups, and multi-specialty group practice networks, which are built around multi-specialty groups. Some network model MCOs incorporate both, and some also permit independent physicians to participate in them.

The IPA Model

At the core of the IPA-type model (Figure 6) is an organization of individual physicians known as an Individual Practice Association (IPA), which may be organized in accordance with a variety of legal structures, among them, not-for-profit corporations, for-profit corporations, partnerships, and associations. Under this model, it is the IPA that contracts with the MCO, in effect permitting individual physicians to participate in HMOs and other managed care products. (Author's note: Discussion of IPA-type MCOs is sometimes confusing because the term "IPA" refers both to a specific type of MCO and to the organization of doctors that contracts with the MCO. For the sake of clarity, this publication will use the term "IPA-type MCO" to refer to the MCO itself, and the term "IPA" to identify that MCO's physician component.)

IPA-type HMOs are attractive to physicians and consumers alike because they typically permit large numbers of physicians to participate in them. However, the larger the IPA, the more difficult it is to manage, given the number of physicians involved and the diffusion of HMO members across a large physician panel. Theoretically, then, an IPA-type HMO should be inherently less efficient than a more tightly structured HMO. While there may be greater potential for better management within more tightly structured models, there are, however, many exceptions to this theory; in fact, some IPA-type HMOs actually perform more effectively than some group or staff model HMOs. However, experts predict that although the more loosely structured MCO models are expected to enjoy a significantly faster growth rate during the early 1990s, the performance and bottom-line successes of more tightly structured models may gradually begin attracting an increased percentage of the market as the decade progresses.

The Direct Contract Model

Discussion of direct contract model MCOs can also be confused by loosely used terminology. As we saw in our discussion of the rapid proliferation of new managed care products, some employers have demonstrated interest in directly contracting with providers for managed care services, eliminating third parties in the process — hence the term "direct contracting." The term "direct contract model MCO," however, refers to a different kind of arrangement.

The term "direct contract model MCO" originally came into being to describe a new form of relationship of physicians to an MCO, one that evolved during the 1980s out of the original IPA-type HMO model. In the 1970s, when the first such IPA-type MCOs were organized, they typically did so by developing two separate corporate entities: one the licensed managed care organization, the other the organization of doctors, or IPA, that contracted with the MCO to provide services to its members. The IPA in turn contracted with each of the physicians who were to participate in it.

> Some IPAs were founded by physicians for the purpose of preserving the status quo, rather than for the purpose of maximizing value.

However, the motives of some physicians in forming IPAs were sometimes mixed. Some IPAs, for example, were founded by physicians for the primary purpose of preserving the status quo, rather than for the purpose of maximizing value. For obvious reasons, such an organization proved to be of limited value in a health care market demanding change. While the leadership of many IPAs recognized the importance of responding to the demands of the marketplace, others were less responsive, and that led to the development of the direct contract model MCO (Figure 7), in which the MCO contracts directly with individual physicians, eliminating the IPA.

The PHO/HPO Model

Physician-Hospital Organization (PHO) or Hospital-Physician Organization (HPO) model MCOs also exist (Figure 8). These have come into being where hospitals and physicians or their medical staffs have joined together through a joint venture structure to create a delivery system that can contract with either MCOs, insurance companies, or directly with employers. However, HPOs and PHOs remain primarily delivery systems, rather than insurance products, as are HMOs, for example.

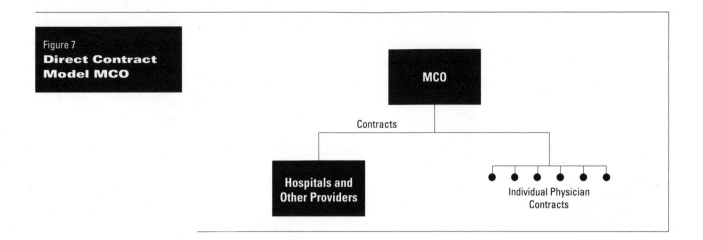

Figure 7
**Direct Contract
Model MCO**

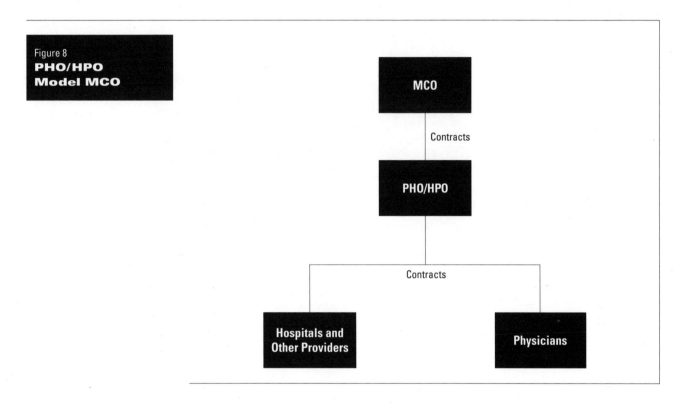

Figure 8
**PHO/HPO
Model MCO**

The Fully-Integrated Delivery System Model

The obvious trend in the development of managed care organizations is the continual blurring and blending of delivery system models for the sake of developing structures through which to successfully deliver a variety of managed care products. It is safe to assume that most managed care organizations will eventually evolve into fully-integrated delivery system models that contain the features of several models. Figure 9 illustrates how such an arrangement might look.

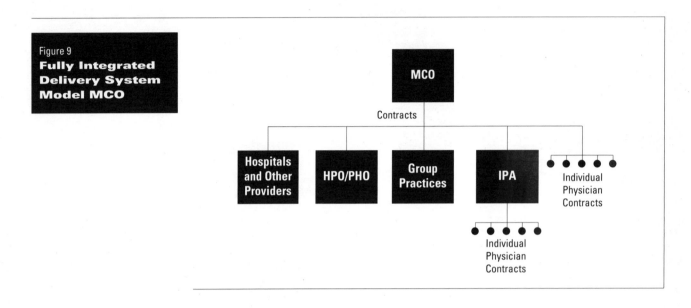

Figure 9
Fully Integrated Delivery System Model MCO

Chapter 2:

The Managed
Care Market

"**M**anaged care market share" is the term used to

describe the percentage of a total national, state, regional, or

local population participating in managed care products. It is

an important term for physicians to understand.

The Physician and Managed Care

For example, Table 1 indicates that as of the end of 1992, HMOs held a market share of 16.1 percent of the total US population, while the PPO market share was 18 percent, for a combined HMO-PPO market share of 34.1 percent. (Managed care market share also may be expressed as a percentage of an insured population, rather than of the total population. In the interest of consistency, market share will be discussed here as a percentage of total population.)

As a general rule, managed care products hold higher market shares in metropolitan markets than in non-metropolitan areas. For example, although HMO market share stood at 16.1 percent as of 1992, it averaged 22 percent in the 30 largest metropolitan areas at the same time. The pattern tends to be reflected at the state level, as well. For example, 18 percent of the population of Minnesota were enrolled in HMOs and 24 percent participated in PPOs, for a statewide combined market share total of 42 percent. In the metropolitan area of Minneapolis, however, the combined managed care market share stood at an estimated 70-80 percent. Among the states, California has for many years led the country in managed care market share, with 77 percent of the state's population participating in managed care products, as of most recently available statistics, 31 percent in HMOs, and 46 percent in PPOs. Indeed, there are some communities in California in which a single HMO has enrolled as much as 60 percent of the total population.

Managed care market share is an important measure to physicians because it represents the percentage of a population that may not be seen by physicians who do not participate in a managed care product. Any physician pondering the implications of that fact may wish to keep in mind that the rapid expansion in managed care of past years has not been the result of some artificial government mandate. Rather, it represents a response to a marketplace demand for control over health care costs and improvements in the quality of care and service.

Table 1
Current HMO and PPO Market Share[1]

	Enrollment/Eligibility[2]	Market Share
HMO	41.4M	16.1%
PPO	45.0M	18.0%
Total HMO and PPO	86.4M	34.1%

[1]Excludes managed fee-for-service.

[2]Source: Group Health Association of America (12/31/92) and American Managed Care and Review Association (12/31/91).

Some critics may point out that managed care has not fulfilled the cost, access, and quality objectives identified when Congress originally passed Public Law 93-222, the Health Maintenance Organization Act of 1973, and to some degree they are right. However, reorganizing the health care industry is an enormously complex challenge. Managed care has been successful enough that it has become the vehicle favored by government policy-makers who seek to implement health system reform, as well as employers and employees. Most of the various health care reform proposals under consideration as this was written would convert the health care industry into a managed care system. As of this writing, the states of Florida and Washington have passed legislation that will implement managed care systems. Other states are considering similar legislation, and it is expected that the federal government will pass legislation implementing a managed care proposal. If enacted, such legislation could spark significant growth in managed care in the US.

Legislation could spark significant growth in managed care in the US.

Whether or not managed care is implemented through government health system reform legislation, managed care will undoubtedly continue to grow in market share as more and more of the general public and employers come to understand the methods used in managed care to reduce the cost of health care.

The managed care industry is still a relatively young one. Accurate statistics on all types of managed care products and organizations are therefore few. However, HMOs have been tracked fairly carefully since the early 1970s, and PPOs since the 1980s. These statistics may offer at least some insights into managed care market trends.

In reviewing these statistics it should be noted that PPO products, by their very nature, do not involve a "locked-in" population. Thus, PPO statistics are cited in terms of those who are eligible to participate, rather than in terms of those who are enrolled.

Table 2 illustrates, by state, the level of HMO enrollment as of July 1, 1992, and PPO eligibility as of January 1, 1990, the latest periods for which these statistics are available. As of December 31, 1992, 546 HMOs were serving a combined enrollment of 38.8 million people nationwide. Of these, approximately 37.2 million were enrolled in "pure" HMOs — that is, those that provide coverage only for a member's use of HMO panel physicians — and 1.6 million in "open-ended" HMOs, those that provide some coverage for use of non-panel physicians. Figures 10 and 11 indicate the growth in the numbers of HMOs and their enrollment from 1980 through 1992. It is interesting to note that although HMO enrollment grew at a steady rate during that time, the number of HMOs in the country peaked at 650 in 1987, then declined to 546 by December 1992.

Table 2

HMO Enrollment and PPO Eligibility by State

	HMO Enrollment[1]	PPO Eligibility[2]
U.S. Total	**37,199,140**	**41,385,000**
1. California	9,732,832	12,800,000
2. New York	3,037,772	2,000,000
3. Massachusetts	1,980,512	1,800,000
4. Florida	1,796,071	500,000
5. Pennsylvania	1,704,317	1,200,000
6. Illinois	1,704,095	1,100,000
7. Michigan	1,518,360	1,300,000
8. Ohio	1,484,779	1,200,000
9. Texas	1,366,130	2,000,000
10. Wisconsin	1,032,093	500,000
11. New Jersey	918,488	1,000,000
12. Maryland	896,561	600,000
13. Minnesota	808,546	500,000
14. Washington	802,404	500,000
15. Oregon	744,354	1,500,000
16. Colorado	724,253	1,900,000
17. Arizona	705,135	600,000
18. Connecticut	641,738	500,000
19. Missouri	547,207	1,000,000
20. North Carolina	372,462	200,000
21. Indiana	356,106	200,000
22. Georgia	333,696	700,000
23. Virginia	322,075	300,000
24. Utah	290,102	400,000
25. Hawaii	256,482	50,000
26. Louisiana	248,144	300,000
27. Kentucky	236,499	800,000
28. New Mexico	236,393	600,000
29. Alabama	216,991	300,000
30. Oklahoma	211,354	1,200,000
31. Tennessee	180,913	1,300,000
32. Kansas	165,237	100,000
33. Nevada	133,689	50,000
34. New Hampshire	126,058	150,000
35. Rhode Island	120,072	300,000
36. Delaware	111,248	20,000
37. Nebraska	107,298	500,000
38. Iowa	107,178	300,000
39. South Carolina	80,741	50,000
40. West Virginia	72,805	400,000
41. Arkansas	65,574	100,000
42. Vermont	53,828	20,000
43. Maine	48,663	15,000
44. Idaho	20,351	10,000
45. Montana	10,731	0
46. North Dakota	6,072	0
District of Columbia	488,594	100,000
Guam	74,137	0
Alaska	0	10,000
Mississippi	0	250,000
South Dakota	0	10,000
Wyoming	0	25,000

[1]Enrollment as of July 1, 1992.

[2]Eligibility as of January 1, 1990

Note: The District of Columbia has been excluded from the state ranking due to the cross-state nature of its enrollment. Guam has been excluded from the rankings as it is not a state. However, enrollment for both D.C. and Guam remain in the U.S. total enrollment figure.

Source: InterStudy, The Competitive Edge, Vol.2, No. 2, 1993

Although the statistics available for PPOs are less well documented than those for HMOs, American Association of Preferred Provider Organizations data indicates that PPOs increased from 115 in 1984 to approximately 800 in 1990. PPOs, of course, came into existence later than HMOs. Therefore, it is not unlikely that the number of these organizations also will peak, perhaps by mid-decade, and then decline, following a normal industry growth curve, with the many players who rush into an industry in its early years gradually shaken out as stronger players demonstrate superior performance. In fact, some experts predict that the number of HMOs in the US may shrink to as few as 200 or less by the end of the decade, although those that survive will be larger than the average HMO currently in operation. Depending upon which version of health care reform is enacted in each state and for the US as a whole, it is also possible that there may be a brief growth spurt of MCOs, which, should it occur, is also likely to eventually follow this trend line.

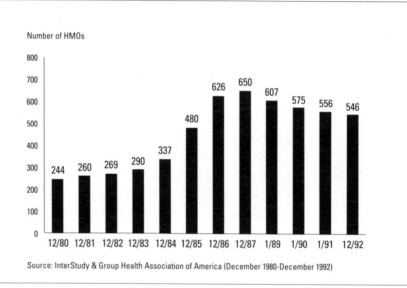

Figure 10
Growth in Number of HMOs
December 1980-December 1992

Number of HMOs

Source: InterStudy & Group Health Association of America (December 1980-December 1992)

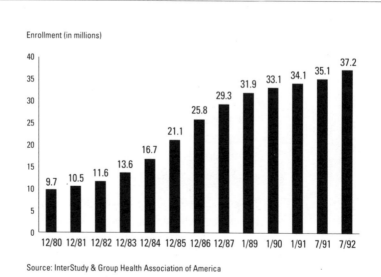

Figure 11
Growth in "Pure" HMO Enrollment
December 1980-July 1992

Enrollment (in millions)

Source: InterStudy & Group Health Association of America

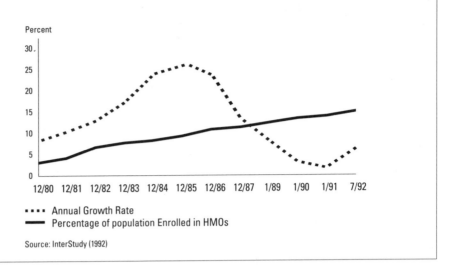

Percent

30
25
20
15
10
5
0

12/80 12/81 12/82 12/83 12/84 12/85 12/86 12/87 1/89 1/90 1/91 7/92

- - - - Annual Growth Rate
——— Percentage of population Enrolled in HMOs

Source: InterStudy (1992)

Figure 12, which charts the annual growth rate of HMOs and the percentage of population enrolled from December 1980 through July 1992, demonstrates another normal industry growth curve: as a market becomes more deeply penetrated, its growth rate tends to slow. The introduction of other managed care products during this time also, of course, has had an impact on the growth of HMOs, especially in some markets. However, it should be noted that the 6.1 percent HMO growth rate that occurred between January 1991 and July 1992 was the highest since 1988. According to the Group Health Association of American, more than half of all active physicians in the US now conduct at least part of their medical practice in association with an HMO.

The Managed Care Consumer

For most managed care products there are, in fact, two managed care consumers: the patient and the patient's employer or some other major purchaser of health care, such as Medicare and Medicaid. Typically, the employer must enter into a group contract with an MCO before the patient even has the option of participating in a managed care product. Thus, there are really two separate points of sale that the MCO must overcome to acquire new members.

According to a 1989 survey by the benefits consulting firm A. Foster Higgins, close to two-thirds of respondent employers offered an HMO option to their employees, a percentage that was greatest among larger employers. No similar statistics are available for PPOs, but the author's experience suggests that PPOs are available to at least the same number of employers, if not more. (Of course, some employers offer the option of several HMOs to their employees, and perhaps one or more PPOs as well, together with a standard indemnity plan. However, some are now beginning to eliminate the indemnity option altogether.)

The federal government, a major purchaser of health care services, has been offering managed care options to federal employees and Medicare beneficiaries since the 1970s, and, as of 1992, more than 25 percent of all federal employees — approximately 2.5 million persons — were enrolled in HMOs. Although only 2.1 million Medicare beneficiaries were enrolled in HMOs in 1992, the number is likely to increase during the 1990s due to federal government policy.

Table 5

Top 25 PPOs Ranked by Number of Eligibles
June 30, 1991

PPO Name/Headquarters	Eligibles[1]
1. Blue Cross Prudent Buyer Plan/Woodland Hills, CA	1,927,198
2. Preferred Provider Network/Berwyn, PA	1,876,250
3. USA Healthnet-Network TX/Phoenix, AZ	1,858,500
4. Community Care Network/San Diego, CA	1,547,358
5. Blue Cross & Blue Shield-Preferred Care/Birmingham, AL	1,505,893
6. Blue Shield Preferred Plan/Blue Shield of CA/San Francisco, CA	1,312,538
7. Blue Cross & Blue Shield of FL Pref. Patient Care/Jacksonville, FL	1,131,413
8. Preferred Health Network/Long Beach, CA	978,850
9. Admar Corp. Med Network/Long Beach, CA	968,753
10. USA Healthnet-Network CA/Phoenix, AZ	943,375
11. Participating Provider Option/Chicago, IL	936,743
12. PPO Alliance/Woodland Hills, CA	920,000
13. Blue Cross & Blue Shield-Preferred Care/Chattanooga, TN	821,135
14. Interplan Corporation/Stockton, CA	652,500
15. USA Healthnet-Network FL/Phoenix, AZ	611,250
16. Blue Cross & Blue Shield-Preferred Care/Indianapolis, IN	557,500
17. Blue Cross & Blue Shield of Missouri/St. Louis, MO	520,878
18. HealthNetwork Inc./Oak Brook, IL	502,500
19. Colorado Preferred Physician Organization/Wheat Ridge, CO	502,500
20. Conservicare/Huntington Beach, CA	500,000
21. National Health Plan Corp./New York, NY	475,000
22. King County Medical Blue Shield/Seattle, WA	453,105
23. USA Healthnet-Network KY/Phoenix, AZ	451,613
24. San Diego PPO/San Diego, CA	400,388
25. MedicalControl/Dallas, TX	400,000

[1]Based on 2.5 eligibles per employee.

Source: SMG Marketing Group, Inc. — Based on a survey of individual reporting PPO plans.

Provider Participation

At the present time, most hospitals in the US have contracts with a variety of managed care organizations, some as many as 50 or more. Half of all physicians in the nation also participate in at least one HMO, and many participate in several, as well as one or more PPO. Although no statistics are available on the number of physicians who participate in PPOs, it is safe to assume an even higher level of participation by physicians in PPOs than in HMOs, given the greater number of PPOs and the fact that many physicians find them more readily acceptable, at least initially, than they do HMOs.

> Half of all physicians in the nation participate in at least one HMO, and many participate in several.

Thus, it is likely that the overwhelming majority of US physicians are already participating in one form of managed care or another. As the decade progresses, and as physicians become more familiar with and experienced in the business of managed care, it is reasonable to assume that managed care results, in terms of changes in utilization patterns and positive impact on the quality of care, will continue to improve.

Managed Care and the Physician

Many factors have been at play that explain the dramatic changes that have been occurring in the demand for hospital and physician services, the growing acceptance of the managed care concept among them. Table 6 illustrates changes in hospital utilization per 1,000 under age 65 population among beneficiaries of indemnity insurance plans and those of managed care organizations as it occurred in the 1970s and as it is currently occurring in the early 1990s. Indeed, with some HMOs planning to virtually eliminate the need for hospitalization except for intensive care, certain procedures, and certain other limited purposes, some HMOs project a utilization rate of fewer than 100 days per 1,000 population within the next 10 to 20 years.

One cause — as well as an effect — of this trend, is the overall movement toward providing as much care as possible in the often less expensive ambulatory setting. As Table 7 illustrates, the trend is expected to have a significant impact on how health care dollars are spent. Theoretically, as the shift from in-patient to ambulatory care occurs, it should result in an overall reduction in the total amount of money spent per patient per year for all health care services, and, in fact, this is usually the case. The implications are clear: in the future, an increasing proportion of the total health care dollar will be spent on physician and other non-hospital services.

Table 6
Indemnity vs. Managed Care Hospital Utilization Patterns

	1970s	1990s
Indemnity Insurance	900-1,000 days/1,000	300-400 days/1,000
Managed Care	500-600 days/1,000	200-300 days/1,000

Table 7
Changes in Percentage of the Health Care Dollar Spent for Hospital vs. Physician and Other Services

1970s	1990s
60%-70% = Hospital	25%-30% = Hospital
30%-40% = Physician and Other	70%-75% = Physician and Other

Although this trend is not likely to result in any windfalls for physicians, it is likely to result in available resources to reimburse physicians who bring real value to the entire health care system. While this bodes well for some physicians, the picture for others is somewhat more clouded, especially for those who fail to respond constructively to the new needs of the market.

> The supply and demand imbalance that already exists between primary care physicians and certain subspecialties can be expected to be exacerbated.

Unfortunately, the supply and demand imbalance that already exists between primary care physicians and certain subspecialties can be expected to be exacerbated. The demand for primary care physicians is increasing disproportionately to the supply. In fact, a shortage of primary care physicians, already acute in some markets, is a major constraint to managed care growth. It is anticipated that this problem will become substantially more severe during the 1990s. In contrast, as the managed care market share increases and as managed care organizations become more tightly managed, the volume of services referred to subspecialists per 1,000 population can be expected to continue to decline.

A look at how the ratio of primary care doctors to subspecialists has already changed in one multi-specialty medical group offers a glimpse into what the future may hold.

In 1972, when a well-known multi-specialty medical group first contemplated pursuing the HMO business, the managed care market share in its community stood at zero. At that time, the group included one part-time true primary care physician, as well as six or seven internists and pediatricians whose practices involved both primary and subspecialty care. All of the other members of its almost 70-doctor staff were subspecialists.

Twenty years later, in 1992, when local managed care market share had increased to 40 percent, slightly more than half of the medical group's patients were participants in managed care products. Its staff had grown from some 70 physicians to more than 200. However, among that staff the ratio of full-time-equivalent primary care physicians to subspecialists had shifted from approximately 1:15 to 1:1.

The dramatic change in the primary care-subspecialist ratio should come as no surprise, however. After all, tightly managed MCOs require most care to be managed by and accessed through a primary care physician. If the primary care physician does that job effectively, patient self-referral to subspecialists will decline.

Indeed, introduction of a primary care patient manager or "gatekeeper", as they are sometimes inappropriately referred to, should eliminate almost all primary care activity in the subspecialist's office. Some studies suggest that primary care comprises as much as 50 percent of some subspecialties' patient volume. In addition, giving the primary care physician the responsibility and authority, as well as the systems support, to manage (or at least monitor) the patient throughout the entire health care delivery system, should result in a reduction in unnecessary referrals and services and will assure a key factor of success: that every referral, admission or service that is necessary is made immediately.

The experience of the one multi-specialty medical group we have looked at is now being replicated in medical groups, academic medical centers, hospital medical staffs, and most other medical communities throughout the country. It is with confidence, therefore, that one can predict that the shortage of primary care physicians will become increasingly acute in the years ahead. This forecast is good news for most primary care physicians, who can expect that their perceived value to society and the health care industry will undoubtedly steadily increase over time. The forecast for certain subspecialty physicians is more clouded. As the demand for their services declines, subspecialists may expect a concomitant decline in perceived value — a perception that is likely to drive their reimbursement closer to that of their primary care colleagues. While debate over the pros and cons of this phenomenon may be heated as competition for increasingly scarce health care dollars intensifies, it is likely that primary care physicians will achieve greater influence and responsibility, and a higher percentage of the health care dollar in the coming years.

The critical question for all physicians, of course, remains not who will receive more patients, contracts, or reimbursement, but, rather, whether their patients are receiving better service and higher quality, more cost-effective health care. All undoubtedly are likely to agree that that will remain the criteria by which managed care will be judged.

Implications for Primary Care Physicians

Obviously, the years ahead are likely to be years of opportunity for primary care physicians. But this opportunity carries with it a corresponding responsibility. Primary care physicians must be able to assure the health care industry that they are well prepared to undertake their role, with adequate preparation in preventive health care, clinical decision-making, cost-effective health care, and the role and responsibility of the physician as case manager. Primary care physicians must be trained in, and become comfortable working within, the framework of a managed care organization. Yet a number of primary care physician residency programs still provide little or no managed care training or experience.

> Primary care physicians must be trained in, and become comfortable working within, the framework of a managed care organization.

The years ahead may offer great opportunity to primary care physicians, but without the appropriate skills and training they will need to thrive in a managed care environment, neither they nor their patients will be well served.

Implications for Subspecialty Physicians

The anticipated shift in demand for subspecialists will undoubtedly be the cause of significant distress for many physicians. Not only will there be substantial competition for patients as a result of decreasing utilization of subspecialty services per 1,000 population, but subspecialists' relationships with primary care physicians will become a much more significant factor in their practice. At the same time, there is likely to be a drop in inappropriate patient self-referrals, enabling subspecialists to focus on their areas of clinical expertise.

The subspecialist's ability to understand how to maximize value in his or her area of specialization can be expected to determine the degree to which he or she will successfully weather the changing environment. Access to information about their own practice patterns, outcomes, and cost, and how these indicators compare to those of their peers — especially those peers who have been objectively identified as achieving superior outcomes — will be essential. Subspecialists who can expect to have the brightest prospects will be those who can put this kind of information to work in their own practices and thereby become standard setters in maximizing quality and patient service while minimizing cost.

> The primary care-subspecialty relationship is likely to evolve in ways that few clinical planners yet anticipate.

A larger role in educating and supporting primary care physicians in diagnosis to assure appropriate and timely referrals is also likely. Indeed, the role of clinician/teacher could become an extremely important component of subspecialty in the future. In fact, the primary care-subspecialty relationship is likely to evolve in ways that few clinical planners yet anticipate.

Chapter 3:

Contracting With an MCO

Much has been written about the virtues and

successes of managed care. Much has been written about its

flaws and failures. Much that has been written is accurate;

some is not. With more than 1,000 managed care organizations

currently in existence in the US, it is not surprising that wide

variations exist among them. As can probably be fairly said of

any large group of organizations, these MCOs range in quality from those that are poorly managed, financially-troubled organizations that provide poor-quality care, to those that are well-managed, soundly financed, and offer the highest quality of care. A physician's decision as to whether to participate in an MCO, or which to join, therefore is not an easy one. Let's consider some of the factors that might go into the decision-making process.

The Promise and the Pitfalls

Overall, many opportunities exist for physicians in managed care, especially those related to its potential to help build or maintain a medical practice through the acquisition of new patients. But it potentially offers other advantages, as well.

First, well-managed MCOs offer the physicians important support services, such as the provision of key patient and practice management information, which can help the physician provide and manage high quality health care in a cost-effective fashion. Some MCOs also offer physicians opportunities to learn or improve certain skills, such as quality management, peer review, team building, teaching, research, and clinical guideline development skills.

The "pros" of managed care are readily apparent. The "cons" tend to be a bit more difficult for physicians to identify.

First, as with any business opportunity, the greatest potential pitfall is lack of real understanding of the opportunity that is being presented. Lack of understanding often leads to surprises after a contract is signed, and surprises in any business arrangement most often mean bad news.

For example, an MCO may never deliver the patients that affiliation with it seems to promise. It may fail to provide the support necessary to effectively manage high quality care. Some MCOs have even been known to cause a degradation in the quality of care and service, or actually to drive up the cost of care, through bad management, poorly conceived systems, and the imposition of unnecessary hassles on physicians and their staffs. And a troubled MCO could mean insufficient reimbursement to physicians, or even none at all.

Fortunately, the competitive pressures of the marketplace are beginning to eliminate MCOs that are unable to document significant improvements in cost and quality, or that are poorly managed and poorly financed. Even so, it may be several years before this process of natural selection is complete.

Weighing Personal Issues

Aside from these larger issues, there are a number of other, more personal considerations that each physician must weigh in evaluating a managed care opportunity. If each MCO has its unique characteristics, certainly that is even more true of each individual physician. Each physician's decision, therefore, must take into consideration the physician's own professional and personal objectives, training and experience, and practice style.

Practice Style

Although some physicians have been successful in the indemnity market without having to be "customer friendly," the managed care industry demands something more. A physician's success in managed care will, to a great degree, be contingent upon the ability to provide prompt, friendly service in a setting that is pleasant and well maintained. This may require substantial training on the part of some physicians' staffs, as well as behavior modification on the part of some physicians. It is not unusual for MCOs to terminate contracts with physicians who fail to learn the importance of good patient relations. Therefore, those who cannot respond to this demand are likely to have a difficult time in the health care marketplace of the 1990s.

> A physician's success in managed care will, to a great degree, be contingent upon the ability to provide prompt, friendly service in a setting that is pleasant and well maintained.

Any physician seeking understanding of how personal practice style can serve as an indicator of success in the managed care environment would do well to review *Managing Health Care: A Teaching Syllabus,* by Doctors Robert Eidus and Samuel W. Warburton (see Bibliography, page 79). In their text, the authors point out that participation in a managed care product requires more than "business as usual" in terms of how the physician communicates with and otherwise relates to managed care patients.

Eidus and Warburton write that physicians practicing in managed care environments "must have a service orientation which includes good communication skills, accessibility, availability, and the ability to work with others." In addition, they "must be comfortable working within an organization...and have good team skills." As they note, HMOs are looking for physicians who can facilitate the effective utilization of resources, physicians who share the philosophy that "more is not always better."

After exploring in depth the major practice style issues related to adaptability to the managed care environment, the authors of this useful work provide a list of questions for physicians to answer in considering managed care options. That list is republished here as Appendix A (page 67).

Ethical Questions

Ideally, the medical ethics that apply in private medical practice should apply equally in the managed care environment. If there were any room for conflict it would most likely lie in the area of resource control, resource utilization, and incentives. The likelihood of such conflict arising in a good MCO is not great, however, and, if it were to occur, the well-run MCO would already have in place protocols for addressing and resolving those conflicts with its physicians.

One way to determine if a potential for conflict exists is simply to talk with physicians who already are affiliated with the MCO in question. Certainly, it is also essential to fully understand the organization's objectives and methods of operation to avoid unpleasant surprises.

The subject of clinical decision-making is, of course, beyond the scope of this publication. However, the authors Eidus and Warburton also offer important insights into ethical issues that may be raised in the managed care setting in a discussion that appears in *The Textbook of Family Practice*, edited by R.E. Rakel, M.D. They write:

> [Critics of managed care organizations] argue that, given the limited resources which we are able to expend on health care, there is no room for corporate profit in the equation. It is also argued that doctors should not be rationers of health care with individual patients. Furthermore, many critics of managed health care feel strongly that incentives to withhold or reduce the intensity of health care to patients is unethical... Advocates of managed health care believe there is enough waste and inefficiency in the health care system that, if any managed care organization, be it for-profit or nonprofit, is able to control the cost of health care, preserve quality, and make health care insurance more affordable and available, then there is a great societal benefit... They feel that HMOs breed competition, which is beneficial. Furthermore, they argue that the behavior of for-profit and nonprofit institutions in terms of attempting to control the bottom line is virtually identical.

In conclusion, Eidus and Warburton say:

> With respect to rationing, most medical directors of HMOs feel that the primary physician should provide medical services for the individual patient up to the level where the maximum medical benefit is achieved. In addition, they argue that the incentive for overutilization in the fee-for-service method of reimbursement is just as harmful as the incentive for underutilization in capitation. Both require utilization and quality management control and the participation of ethical physicians.

Some experts express this issue in the context of the relationship between the quantity of medical services and clinical outcomes, as did Dr. Donald Schaller, founder of one of the leading MCOs in the Southwest, in remarks to the September 1991 American Academy of Family Physicians' Scientific Assembly, in which he described a "Plateau of Comparable Outcomes" (see Figure 13).

Figure 13 suggests that there is an optimal point (B) at which the appropriate quantity of services has been provided, beyond which there is little or no improvement in clinical outcome. At that point, the physician begins to feel substantial pressure from the patient to continue to provide or prescribe more services. Simultaneously, the physician is increasingly being asked to control costs. It is only with a well-designed information system that physicians can begin to know when they are approaching or exceeding point B. That same information can be used for a variety of purposes, including the support of the physician's clinical decisions, should a subsequent question or issue arise. At point C, outcomes begin to degenerate due to iatrogenic and related factors.

Debate over ethical issues like these undoubtedly will continue. Clearly, each MCO must address these issues successfully in order to survive and prosper.

Figure 13
**Plateau of
Comparable
Outcomes**

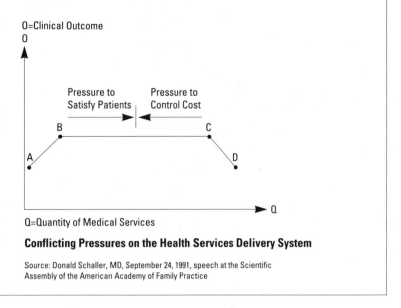

Conflicting Pressures on the Health Services Delivery System

Source: Donald Schaller, MD, September 24, 1991, speech at the Scientific
Assembly of the American Academy of Family Practice

Business Objectives

Participation in managed care products can be a key marketing tool through which physicians can reach not only those individuals insured through an HMO and other managed care coverage, but also those covered under employer self-insured plans, Medicare and Medicaid, and other such mechanisms. The value of this potential tool will, of course, depend upon each physician's personal circumstances. The physician whose retirement is nearing may, after all, have substantially different business objectives from those of one who has recently completed a residency, or is at mid-career.

Any physician who intends to remain in practice throughout the 1990s, however, would be wise to develop some projections of how the local health care market will be shared by the year 2000, starting with current local market share statistics, then relating those statistics to personal revenue goals. In a market where the managed care market share is growing, the dictates of prudent practice management would suggest that the percentage of the physician's revenues deriving from managed care patients be at least equal to, if not slightly greater than, the area's total managed care market share. Substantial declines in a physician's managed care market share behind the areawide managed care market share are likely to leave the physician vulnerable to erosion of the practice's patient base.

> Substantial declines in a physician's managed care market share behind the areawide managed care market share are likely to leave the physician vulnerable to erosion of the practice's patient base.

Establishing specific goals will depend upon the volume and percentage of a practice that each physician wishes to allocate to managed care. That determination will, in turn, depend upon overall practice objectives regarding volume and growth.

Once the current managed care market share for the area has been determined, the next step in this process is to arrive at some rough estimates of managed care growth for the next five to 10 years. If, for example, the current managed care market share is 15 percent and it is reasonable to predict growth to 30 or 40 percent by the end of the decade, then it is possible to estimate the percentage of a practice that will have to be derived from managed care in order to retain a patient base appropriate to achieving personal business goals. Therefore, if 15 percent of a practice is derived from managed care when the current local managed care market share is also 15 percent, then the physician who expects a 30 to 40 percent growth in local market share would need to achieve managed care practice growth to the same percentage (all other things being equal) within the same time frame. Those interested in practice expansion may establish even higher percentage goals.

Once these goals are translated into projected numbers of managed care patients, patient visits, and other key practice management statistics, the data can be used as the basis for estimating the number of managed care contracts that need to be pursued to achieve established goals.

Finding the Right Fit

Even those physicians who are sure they want to participate in managed care have another choice to make: what kind of managed care arrangement is right for you?

Each model suggests certain pros and cons that only the individual physician can balance. For example, for those who already are in a group practice, the group or network model is likely to be more compatible with established modes of operation. To those who prefer solo practice, a PHO or IPA-type MCO may offer opportunities such as participation in quality management systems that might not otherwise be available.

However, it is important to emphasize that the pros and cons of participating in an MCO relate not so much to model types as to the management style and clinical quality of the MCO under consideration, the terms and conditions of its standard provider contracts, and the support services it will supply. In the final analysis, it is those things that will make a difference not only in whether or not the MCO itself is successful, but also in whether or not an individual physician is likely to find success within its structure.

Preparing to Negotiate

It would probably require a publication much thicker than this one to address all of the issues raised in a comprehensive discussion of contracts between physicians and managed care organizations. Nonetheless, no discussion of managed care would be complete without at least touching upon some of the issues typically raised when a physician contemplates entering into a managed care contract.

It is safe to say that one of the most important items to be covered in physician-MCO contract negotiations is the question of which services are and are not covered by the contract. Every physician must fully understand, in the most specific terms, exactly what services he or she is obligated to provide under the contract. All such services should be cited in the contract, and, in many cases, identified by procedure code.

> Every physician must fully understand, in the most specific terms, exactly what services he or she is obligated to provide under the contract.

Policies regarding noncovered services also must be clearly articulated. The fact that an MCO does not cover a particular service does not necessary mean that the physician cannot or should not provide that service to one of its members if it is medically necessary to do so. It is, however, important to clarify during negotiations how reimbursement for such services will be handled. Nor should there be any ambiguity about how compensation is determined. If reimbursement for all services provided is to be on a capitation basis, precise definitions of those services is essential. Because subspecialists are most likely to be reimbursed on a fee-for-service basis, the exact variations on compensation must be spelled out.

Other kinds of issues that need to be addressed by primary care physicians include how coverage is to be provided during night and weekend hours and over vacations and whether the physician will be permitted to close his or her practice to new managed care patients if it reaches capacity. If payment is to be on a capitation basis, the contract should also address how capitation rate changes will be handled in the event of changes in benefits or the development of new technology that might result in changes in services.

In addition to these general guidelines, a "Basic Managed Care Contract Issues, Terms, and Conditions Checklist" is provided in Table 8. The checklist outlines the issues that, at a minimum, need to be addressed in the negotiating process. In addition, any physician who lacks experience in contract negotiation or the business of managed care is strongly urged to seek the advice of qualified experts before entering into any such agreement.

Assessing the Environment

Many important clues to what a physician-MCO relationship will be can be found in the pre-negotiation and negotiation stages of contract development. Discussions should be forthright and the MCO should demonstrate understanding and concern about any legitimate issues raised by the physician. The MCO that is not attentive to physician concerns in this courtship phase is not likely to be more so once the honeymoon is over.

Good information is absolutely essential to the decision-making process. Therefore, it is critical that timely, adequate, and accurate reports by made available by the MCO. Primary care physicians, for example, should receive reports that detail both current month and year-to-date activities, as well as information on actual performance compared to budget and peers for their panel of patients. Similarly, subspecialists should ultimately be given information regarding their practice patterns, outcomes, and cost, compared to a predetermined standard and adjusted for severity and intensity. In addition to making reports available, the MCO should be willing to attach sample reports to the contract to establish its obligation to the physician.

Table 8

Basic Managed Care Contract Issues, Terms and Conditions Checklist

I. Basic Issues

- [ ] Negotiating strategies
- [ ] How many managed care patients do you need/want each year for the next 10 years?
- [ ] How many managed care contracts are feasible/ necessary to reach your patient volume and managed care percentage targets?
- [ ] Case management/gatekeeper requirements
- [ ] How many primary care physicians are already included in the MCO panel?
- [ ] Current and projected "mix" of MCO members/ enrollees (e.g., age, sex, commercial, Medicare, Medicaid, etc.)
- [ ] Degree of specialist control and general influence over the MCO's policies and procedures (i.e., governance and committee structure)
- [ ] Participating hospitals, specialists, and ancillary providers
- [ ] Utilization management and quality management systems, procedures and support
- [ ] Practice management support supplied by MCO
- [ ] Billing and administrative requirements
- [ ] Management information system and monthly reports to primary care physicians
- [ ] Exclusivity requirements
- [ ] MCO solvency/viability and general reputation and commitment to quality
- [ ] Compensation:
  - _ Methodology
    Fee-for-service
    Discounted fee-for-service/fee schedule
    Risk:
       Fee-for-service with a withhold
       Primary care capitation
       Physician and ancillary services capitation
       Physician, ancillary services, and all other physician services capitation
       All health care services capitation
  - _ Balance billing limitation and hold harmless provision
  - _ Coordination of benefits
  - _ Risk/bonus pools specifics
  - _ Retroactive additions and deletions of eligible members
  - _ Employer audits of MCO and provider records
  - _ Denial of payment conditions
  - _ Timely billing and claims payment requirements
  - _ Rate increases (premium and physician reimbursement)
  - _ Copying costs (Who is responsible?)
  - _ Insolvency protection for physician
  - _ Financial statements/reporting
  - _ Cognitive skills reimbursement
  - _ Adverse selection
  - _ Incentives versus sanctions
  - _ Adequacy of primary care physician capitation
  - _ Actuarial soundness of premium rates
  - _ Timeliness of payment
  - _ "Escalator" clauses
  - _ Case management reimbursement factor (e.g., monthly fee)
  - _ Reimbursement "ratcheting"
  - _ Physician incentive system (How does it work?)
  - _ Copayments, coinsurance, and deductibles
  - _ Noncovered services (Who pays for?)
  - _ Surcharges
  - _ Stop loss provisions/reinsurance
  - _ Limitations for major disaster or epidemic, labor disputes

II. Basic Terms and Conditions

- [ ] Provision of services by physician
  - _ List of covered services
  - _ Standards of care
  - _ Referrals
  - _ Hospitalization
  - _ Nondiscrimination of members in physician's practice
  - _ Access of patients to physician
  - _ Medical records requirements
  - _ Practice sites
  - _ Signs required in physician's office
  - _ Compliance with MCO rules and regulations
  - _ Exclusivity requirements
  - _ Coordination of benefits (COB) procedures
  - _ Release of medical records and confidentiality
  - _ Mandatory audits by MCO or its agent
  - _ Indemnification and hold harmless provision
  - _ Professional liability insurance requirements
  - _ General liability insurance requirements
- [ ] Administrative responsibilities of MCO
  - _ Monthly patient/member activity and cost reports to physician
  - _ Eligibility reporting
  - _ Payment/payment in full
  - _ Utilization review and quality assurance
  - _ Patient transfers out of PCP panel upon request
  - _ Independent contractor provision
  - _ Grievance procedures
  - _ Site evaluations
  - _ Advertising and marketing
  - _ Data support
  - _ Licenses and permits
  - _ Confidentiality
- [ ] Other basic terms and conditions
  - _ Renegotiation language
  - _ Mutual indemnification
  - _ Mutual insurance requirements
  - _ Conflicts of interest disclosure requirements
  - _ Term, termination, and default
    Term of contract
    Termination provisions (who, when, how)
    For cause
    No fault
    Notification
    Extension
    Removal of participating provider
  - _ Continuing education requirements
  - _ Hospital privileges requirements
  - _ General provisions
    Waiver
    Entire agreement
    Record maintenance
    Severability of contract
    Amendments to contract
    Governing law
    Successor and assignments
    Notices
    Disputes/Arbitration
  - _ Confidentiality
    Mutual responsibility
    Patient records
    Utilization data
    Quality improvement
    Statutory requirements

Other important matters that should be explored include:

- How the MCO will orient physicians and staff to administrative procedures, and whether it will provide an operations manual for their office.

- Whether there will be access to timely and accurate eligibility information so that physician and staff can easily determine if a patient is currently eligible for MCO benefits.

- Which hospitals, physicians, and ancillary providers are participating in the MCO.

- The prospects for adverse selection, particularly for the physician who receives payment on a capitation basis and who specializes in certain procedures.

- Options available to the physician for dealing with a noncompliant or abusive patient.

- Utilization and quality management system requirements, mandatory audits, and related requirements.

Defining Your Position

Successful negotiations of all kinds require the parties to be clear about their objectives. Nowhere is that more true than in the negotiation of a physician-MCO contract. Physicians typically participate in managed care for two primary reasons: preservation or expansion of their patient base, and revenue protection or expansion. Determining specific business objectives, therefore, is an essential first step in contract negotiation.

> Determining specific business objectives is an essential first step in contract negotiation.

Physicians can also maximize their negotiating ability by accurately assessing those factors that can affect their position, such as the competitive situation, their particular expertise, and so on. Although an individual physician is not likely to have as much bargaining power as a group of physicians, some physicians will have more leverage than others, depending on their specialty, location, and reputation.

Exclusivity

Exclusivity also can be an issue that arises in the negotiating process. It is not unusual for an MCO to request an exclusive relationship — that is, one in which the physician promises not to contract with any other MCO. However, physicians should be aware that it is rarely feasible to guarantee exclusivity to only one MCO unless that MCO is capable of providing all the managed care business volume that the physician desires.

In addition, while exclusive relationships usually are legal, in some circumstances they may not be, as in the case of an MCO with a very large market share or one in which the physician is the only provider of certain services in a particular market. For that reason, physicians should consult their attorneys before requesting or promising exclusivity.

Exclusive arrangements are expected to become more common during the present decade, as relationships between MCOs and physicians become more tightly knit. However, the degree to which exclusivity is an issue is likely to vary substantially from one market to another, depending upon the local managed care market share. It is also an issue that is most likely to affect primary care physicians because MCOs typically differentiate among themselves based on their primary care physician network.

Understanding and Evaluating Capitation

In the past, many physicians viewed managed care as, at best, a necessary evil. Today, attitudes are changing. Some physicians may never participate in managed care, either because they are likely to retire before market factors make it imperative for them to do so, or because they believe they can carve out a market niche of their own. However, "niche" providers are becoming increasingly rare. The likelihood is that most physicians now in or entering practice will need to participate in managed care during their practice lifetimes, and for many of them it will constitute a significant part of their practice.

The economic consequences of that fact usually begin to make themselves felt once 20 to 25 percent of a practice is derived from the managed care segment of the market. Once that level has been achieved, the economics of the situation become significant enough to warrant close attention to the financial impact of the physician's relationship with MCOs. It is therefore essential to understand the kinds of financial arrangements that a physician-MCO relationship may involve, and their likely impact, long before a practice reaches that level of managed care activity.

> Capitation is used primarily to reimburse primary care physicians, multi-specialty group practices and integrated health care systems.

In introducing the assembly line concept to American industry in the early 1900s, Henry Ford sought a way of encouraging employees to produce a higher volume of output, and found it in the piecework compensation system. The same kind of incentive has operated in the health care industry for years under the banner of fee-for-service compensation. Critics of fee-for-service compensation point out that the incentives inherent in it encourage providers not only to increase fees but also to produce a maximum number of services in order to maximize revenue.

The primary business objective of most MCOs is to produce a service or set of services that offers maximum value to its customers, who perceive value in terms of improved health care and service, and controlled costs. One of the things an MCO must achieve to satisfy its customers — managed utilization — conflicts directly with an incentive system that encourages maximization of revenues through the provision of more services. As a purchaser of health care, a typical employer is interested not so much in the cost of a single physician visit or hospital day, but primarily in the total cost of health care per employee per year. To create the same bottom-line perspective among providers, many MCOs have implemented a reimbursement system known as capitation.

To date, capitation has been applied almost exclusively to primary care physicians, multi-specialty group practices, fully-integrated health care systems, and certain services, such as prescription drugs and laboratory and mental health services. Because capitation requires relating a specific panel of patients to a specific physician, subspecialists, with few exceptions, are still most commonly paid on the basis of some variation of the fee-for-service method. Although some MCOs currently are experimenting with capitation in a few subspecialties, such as orthopedics and mental health, it usually is not feasible to capitate subspecialists. For the same reason, few of certain types of managed care organizations — PPOs, for example — use capitation for reimbursing physicians.

As Figure 14 demonstrates, in 1991 72 percent of HMOs reimbursed their primary care physicians on a capitation basis. But not all HMOs rely on capitation, and even those that do so may use it in conjunction with other payment methods; Tables 9 and 10 illustrate the degree to which other methods are used. These statistics, of course, relate to HMOs only. PPOs and other forms of MCOs are much more likely to rely on noncapitated methods of reimbursement as a result of their open-ended nature, which tends to preclude accurate calculation of capitation rates.

Capitation is a method of payment under which providers are reimbursed at a fixed amount per MCO member per month — in other words, per capita. As such, it represents a significant paradigm shift in the basic economics of medical practice, one under which the focus changes from how much the physician will be paid, as is the case in the provision of fee-for-service care, to how much it will cost the physician to provide the services specified in the capitation agreement.

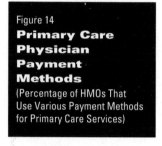

Figure 14
Primary Care Physician Payment Methods
(Percentage of HMOs That Use Various Payment Methods for Primary Care Services)

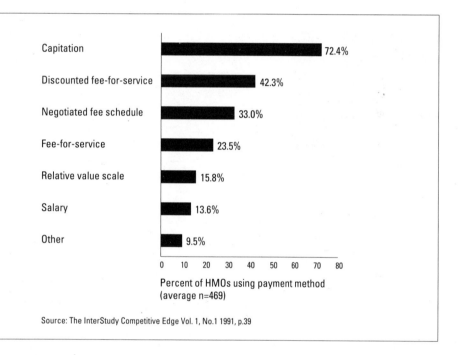

Source: The InterStudy Competitive Edge Vol. 1, No.1 1991, p.39

	Staff (n=37)	Group (n=46)	Network (n=47)	IPA (n=302)	Mixed (n=38)
Capitation	45.9%	89.1%	85.1%	68.0%	97.4%
Discounted fee-for-service	21.6	17.4	53.2	48.5	29.7
Negotiated fee schedule	21.6	15.2	27.7	38.9	26.3
Fee-for-service	24.3	13.0	27.7	26.2	8.1
Relative value scale	0.0	2.2	14.9	21.0	8.1
Salary	94.6	8.7	8.5	2.0	39.5
Other	2.7	17.4	10.6	9.5	5.3

Source: The Interstudy Competitive Edge, Vol. 1 No. 2, Excelsior, MN, 1992.

	Northeast (n=103)	South (n=136)	Midwest (n=136)	West (n=92)
Capitation	68.0%	77.9%	75.7%	65.6%
Discounted fee-for-service	37.9	33.8	47.8	53.3
Negotiated fee schedule	30.4	32.8	34.1	35.9
Fee-for-service	24.5	27.9	20.6	20.9
Relative value scale	12.6	10.4	13.3	30.8
Salary	18.4	10.3	11.9	15.2
Other	11.7	10.1	7.4	9.8

Source: The Interstudy Competitive Edge, Vol. 1 No. 2, Excelsior, MN, 1992.

Because there have been many examples of capitation reimbursement that have placed physicians at undue risk and caused economic hardship, many physicians respond negatively to the very term. It should be noted, however, that there are also many examples of capitation arrangements that are quite adequate, if not quite profitable, for physicians who understand the concept and know how to manage patients effectively.

Limiting Risk

The physician's risk under capitation can — and should be — evaluated, managed, and limited by the physician and the MCO. Where risk does exist in a properly structured primary care physician capitation rate, it is related primarily to the amount of time that will be required for the physician to provide high quality health care to MCO patients. The obvious corollary to this rule is that the physician therefore must be very careful in the use of time, given that it is an extremely limited commodity. It is also important to be careful of capitation contracts that place the physician at risk for services provided outside the office, unless those services are included as part of an overall MCO incentive system, which spreads part of this risk among other participating physicians. Where capitation is used to reimburse a multi-specialty group practice or integrated health system, the scope of services for which the group is at risk increases substantially.

It is also essential to understand exactly what services are included in a capitation rate, regardless of whether capitation applies only to services provided by the individual physician or is more broadly based. Additional risk is not necessarily undesirable, however, depending on how the risk is structured and whether the physician has a reasonable opportunity to manage that risk.

> There are indeed ways of structuring capitation rates that can be extremely attractive to the physician.

There are indeed ways of structuring capitation rates that can be extremely attractive to the physician, and it is these arrangements that need to be understood and sought out. While the uninitiated may view all capitation rates, no matter how structured, as economically disadvantageous, in fact there are arrangements that may result in a more favorable economic outcome than payment on a fee-for-service basis.

The subject of capitation is discussed in depth in a paper entitled "Capitation in IPA-Type HMOs," published by the American Academy of Family Practice.* The following general rules also apply:

- Learn how to evaluate a capitation rate and, if possible, equate it to fee-for-service revenue. For example, if a physician's practice consists of 2,000 patients, and if capitation reimbursement were $8.00 per patient per month, the result would be a gross annual income of $192,000. Admittedly a crude measure in that it does not take variables such as patient mix into account, this conversion process at least provides some familiar benchmarks against which a capitation rate can be measured.

- Be absolutely clear about what specific services are included in the capitation rate, the anticipated frequency in terms of units of service per member per month, and the estimated unit cost for each of those services. These are basic actuarial calculations that the MCO should already have developed, and which it should be willing to share so that physicians can evaluate the adequacy of the capitation rate. It is impossible to evaluate the adequacy of a capitation rate until both the services to be included and the population to be served have been precisely identified.

- Talk with other physicians who have experience with the MCO under consideration. They should be able to provide insight into the adequacy of physician support services and other operational issues.

- In addition to the basic services included in the capitation rate, it is becoming increasingly common for MCOs to add a factor for "cognitive skills" and/or "case management" for primary care physicians in amounts ranging, at this writing, from 50 cents to $2.00 or more per member per month. As the value of the patient manager's cognitive skills increases, it is likely that this line item in the capitation rate, or the unit cost projections contained in the capitation rate, or both, will likewise increase.

*"Capitation in IPA-Type HMOs" is available from AAFP, 8880 Ward Pkwy, Kansas City, MO 64114

One word of caution. Capitation reimbursement arrangements rely upon the law of averages. Therefore, it is unlikely that the financial outcome of such an arrangement will be favorable to the physician if the number of patients for whom capitation payments are received is not of sufficient size. The impact of just one or two patients who demand an inordinate amount of the physician's time can be significant when the panel is small. According to most experts, the long-term economic outlook under a capitation reimbursement plan for a solo primary care physician is not likely to be favorable unless the capitated panel grows to at least 250 to 300 MCO members.

The broader the scope of provider services available in the practice (eg, solo, multi-specialty, Integrated Health System), the broader the capitation (ie, the scope of services included) can be, because more services can be managed by the practice. Age and sex variations in capitation rates also have to be taken into consideration because of the predictably higher use rates of certain components of a patient panel.

The coming years are likely to see the development of more capitation-like reimbursement systems as the managed care industry becomes more sophisticated in developing equitable capitation rates and in providing capitated physicians with the management tools through which they can succeed in this kind of reimbursement program. Therefore, understanding how to make capitation arrangements work in their favor should be a basic survival strategy for all physicians.

The Incentive Chain

Today, the incentives that operate at the primary care physician level of an MCO provider are an important foundation of the entire system. However, incentives also must be created for the rest of the delivery system to encourage the production of value-based health care services. If managed care goals are to be achieved, it makes little sense to create incentives for the primary care physician and not for the subspecialists, hospitals, ancillary providers, and others who complete the MCO delivery system. As a result, MCOs develop comprehensive provider incentive systems which frequently are based on a series of risk pools (eg, primary care, subspecialty, hospital, etc), withholds — that is, a percentage of compensation that is withheld and paid only if utilization goals are met — and bonuses. However, these provider incentive systems sometimes are extremely complex and difficult to evaluate.

Nonetheless, establishing a consistent flow of incentives from purchaser through the MCO to the provider is essential to a successful managed care effort. It is not surprising that analyses of MCOs that have encountered financial difficulties often identify a break in that chain of incentives. Figure 15 illustrates how such a break may occur.

In the scenario illustrated by Figure 15, primary care physician (PCP) #3 enjoys the same economic incentives as does the IPA or group practice with which the physician has a contractual or employment relationship. Similarly, the IPA/group practice experiences the same economic incentives as the MCO, which in turn is reimbursed on the basis of a per capita calculation. In this arrangement, the economic incentives flow consistently throughout.

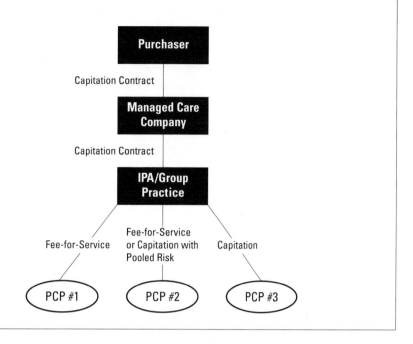

Figure 15
**Provider
Incentive Flow**

PCP #1, however, is being reimbursed on a fee-for-service basis, and thus is inherently in conflict with the incentives that drive the other parties. PCP #2, if reimbursed on a fee-for-service basis with some pooled risk, still is driven by contradictory incentives, although the pooling of risk may bring incentives into closer harmony. If PCP #2 were compensated on a capitation basis, with some pooled risk among peers, a more reliably consistent incentive flow could be achieved.

Toward that end, during the late 1980s an approach to grouping independent primary care physicians became quite popular among a number of MCOs. This approach provides some of the safety in numbers that can be found within a formal primary care group practice. Although variations in the arrangements exist, grouping basically involves identifying a limited number of physicians — typically, six to 12 — who are familiar with each other's practice patterns, standards of care, and so on, and who are comfortable sharing some risk on a limited basis. Although making such an arrangement work usually requires a number of issues to be addressed and resolved, it has proven a successful vehicle by which many independent primary care physicians have been able to gain access to some of the economic advantages of formal group practices. In fact, PCP groupings that have operated for several years tend to evolve into more formalized group practice structures as the physicians involved become aware of the advantages of the arrangement to themselves.

> PCP groupings that have operated for several years tend to evolve into more formalized group practice structures as the physicians involved become aware of the advantages of the arrangements to themselves.

Although variations on the fee-for-service method remain the most popular approach for reimbursing subspecialists, some are paid on a global fee-per-procedure basis, as in the case of obstetricians who are paid a fee-per-procedure for each delivery. Most MCOs attempt to provide incentives to subspecialists through pool arrangements. This is a weak and sometimes dysfunctional incentive design at best, but unless physicians are part of a larger entity that can support them in the delivery of care and the assumption and management of risk for that care, such as a large group practice, there appear to be few, if any, alternatives to this less than ideal approach.

Examining Essential Support Systems

The adequacy of reimbursement is not the only essential issue that must be addressed in assessing a possible relationship with an MCO. No physician can effectively manage care without certain management tools that must be provided by the MCO. Because primary care physicians have significant responsibility for managing MCO members' care, their support requirements tend to be greater than those of subspecialists. They include:

- Monthly reports on the activity of each PCP's entire patient panel for the current month and year-to-date, providing information on all services received, including subspecialty, hospital, ancillary, and pharmacy services. The importance of these tools cannot be overemphasized. Any MCO that is unable or unwilling to provide these essential tools is best avoided.

- Reports that identify specific processes and outcomes for specific diagnoses, adjusted to take severity into account, for use in comparing various subspecialists by procedure. This information is also vital for subspecialists.

In addition, both primary care physicians and subspecialists need the following:

- Assistance in reviewing and interpreting reports.

- Assistance in accessing hospitals, laboratories, pharmacies, and other providers.

- Effective and streamlined utilization management procedures and systems that assist and support rather than hinder physicians in performing their role as patient managers or referred physicians.

- Effective quality management procedures and systems that aid the physician in measuring and monitoring the quality of the entire system, as well the physician's own practice.

- Clinical support in areas such as automated laboratory reporting, linkages to hospital medical records systems, automated treatment protocols and guidelines, and so on.

- Practice management support, such as assistance in preparation and processing of claims, accessing clinical data bases and medical records through automated systems, and basic office management, including providing access to shared purchasing, payroll, and billing services.

- Educational assistance in key clinical areas and in the development of effective practice patterns and styles.

- Systems that permit timely and effective communications with MCO enrollees and other providers on such essential matters as changes in policies, procedures, and benefit eligibility.

The 1990s undoubtedly will see significant improvements in many of these tools. For example, paperless claims systems were already the subject of active experimentation as the decade began and are expected to become industry standards by its end, eliminating the need for physicians' offices to deal with paperwork to process a claim. Such a system would also permit the MCO to immediately accrue claims expenses within its accounting system. The same instant data entry can be achieved with basic encounter information if a provider is paid on a capitation basis and therefore does not ordinarily submit claims.

In the meantime, it is important to remember that the managed care industry is still very much in a developmental phase. Some of these tools may not now be as highly developed in a given MCO as they are likely to be by the end of the decade. The important question, then, may not be whether all these tools are in place at the moment, but whether the organization can demonstrate its commitment to developing them.

> The important question, then, may not be whether all these tools are in place at the moment, but whether the organization can demonstrate its commitment to developing them.

Quality Management

Although they may initially have different business objectives, there can be no question that both physicians and managed care organizations should share the same objective when it comes to the quality of health care: both should desire to deliver the highest quality care possible. If there is any room for conflict, it should only be over questions regarding how quality is defined, measured, and managed.

In the 1970s and 1980s, when questions regarding the quality of health care first emerged as an issue and quality assurance became an important topic of discussion, the terminology then current suggested that it was adequate to simply "assure," on a retrospective basis, that high quality health care was being provided. Toward the end of the 1980s, the term "quality assurance" gradually came to be replaced by "quality management," a term that refers to the basic systems, policies, and procedures that each MCO must develop and implement as part of its overall health care delivery system. As the replacement of the term "quality assurance" by "quality management" suggests, MCOs, and therefore their participating physicians, now are being called upon to become much more aggressive in prospectively managing the quality of the services they provide.

To explain the distinction between these two concepts, some physician leaders in the managed care industry have observed that utilization management involves doing *just* the right thing, while quality management involves doing *all* the right things. Supporting the on-going development and operation of these systems will require a significant investment on the part of MCOs in quality management systems that will maximize the quality, outcomes, and service provided while minimizing total costs per member per month and year.

Writing in *Managed Health Care: A Teaching Syllabus,* Eidus and Warburton identify three elements of a quality management system:

1. *Structure* — that is, how the health care delivery system is organized in terms of its number of primary and subspecialty care physicians per 1,000 members, number of hospital beds available per 1,000 members, the credentials of its providers, and so on.

2. *Process* — the mechanisms by which patients receive care, including the appropriateness and effectiveness of MCO policies and procedures (eg, appointment and office waiting times, time spent with the patient, medical record documentation, compliance with practice guidelines, etc).

3. *Outcome* — The measuring of an objective indicator of the health of an individual or population (eg, percent of newly diagnosed breast cancers that are Stage I or Stage II, incidence of childhood illnesses preventable by immunization, incidence of low birth weight in newborns, etc).

MCO quality management systems need instruments of measurement and a means of evaluating and applying the information produced by those instruments. In addition to the analysis of outcomes, Eidus and Warburton discuss the following means of assessing clinical and patient service quality:

- Member satisfaction questionnaires
- Member transfer rates
- Member termination rates
- Focused chart audits
- Grievances
- Generic screen audits
- Provider credentials
- Review of sanctions against providers
- Pharmacy data regarding unusual prescribing patterns
- Utilization data (with special emphasis on underutilization)
- Appropriateness of procedures that are often underutilized (ie, C-section, hysterectomy, carotid endartectomy)

> An effective quality management system will include the process of credentialing and recredentialing participating physicians.

Figure 16 presents the results of a survey conducted in 1990 by Interstudy, an HMO research group based in Minneapolis. At least half of the 479 responding HMOs reported using all of the top seven quality control measures listed.

An effective quality management system will include the process of credentialing and re-credentialing participating physicians. This is an area that has been neglected by some MCOs that have sought to enhance their appeal to potential beneficiaries by maximizing the number of physicians on their panels, believing the availability of a wide choice of providers to be necessary to gaining acceptance and market share. As a result, these MCOs have placed a lower priority on assuring that the physicians on their panels manage the cost and quality of service effectively.

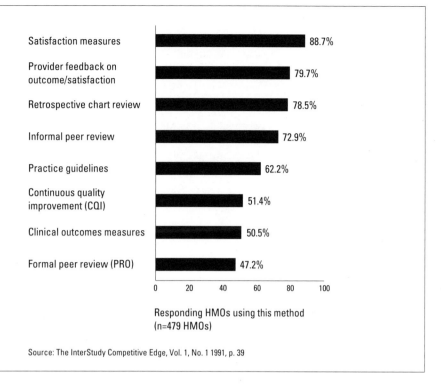

Figure 16
HMO Quality Control Measures

Measure	%
Satisfaction measures	88.7%
Provider feedback on outcome/satisfaction	79.7%
Retrospective chart review	78.5%
Informal peer review	72.9%
Practice guidelines	62.2%
Continuous quality improvement (CQI)	51.4%
Clinical outcomes measures	50.5%
Formal peer review (PRO)	47.2%

Responding HMOs using this method
(n=479 HMOs)

Source: The InterStudy Competitive Edge, Vol. 1, No. 1 1991, p. 39

Figure 17
Components of a Comprehensive Managed Care Organization Quality Management System

Quality Management System		
Clinical Quality	Service Quality	Management and Systems Quality

However, market pressures on HMOs for objective proof of the quality of care and services they provide during the 1990s can be expected to cause MCOs to become more selective about the physicians on their panels, and therefore MCOs will place greater emphasis on credentialing and recredentialing participating physicians. The market pressures will be generated by greater acceptance of managed care, a higher degree of competition over cost, and greater beneficiary interest in the quality of care provided by an MCO panel. MCOs will not be able to afford participating physicians who do not manage cost and quality effectively.

Figure 17 illustrates the three components that are essential to a comprehensive MCO quality management system. Their interdependency cannot be overemphasized. Obviously, the quality of clinical services will be directly affected by the quality of the physicians providing those services; it will also be either enhanced or undermined by the MCO's management and systems. The primary factors that patients consider in determining the quality of the medical care they receive usually are such things as its convenience to them, the kind of attention they receive, the friendliness of office staff, the willingness of staff members to answer questions, and so on. Thus all three components —clinical, service, management and systems — must be addressed by the MCO's quality management system. Physicians are well advised to thoroughly investigate these systems in the process of making decisions about which MCOs to affiliate with over the long term.

Depending upon the models on which they are based, MCOs may differ substantially in their approach to and ability to monitor and manage clinical and service quality. For example, staff model HMOs, in which all physicians are employed directly by the HMO and located within the HMO's facilities, present an environment that differs substantially from that of an IPA-model HMO, whose individual participating physicians may be distributed throughout a large geographic region. Staff model HMOs have greater control over the physicians on their panels than do IPA-model HMOs, and they also have greater control over their office staffs and premises. It is therefore easier for a staff model HMO to monitor and manage quality than it is for an IPA-model HMO, which relies on a panel of independent, autonomous physicians that own their offices and control their own office staffs. As a result, staff model HMOs have a theoretical competitive advantage over other models. However, this advantage is not insuperable if IPA-model physicians are attentive to and cooperative with efforts by the HMO to help physicians monitor and manage clinical quality and service quality.

> MCOs may differ substantially in their approach to and ability to monitor and manage clinical and service quality.

A number of software firms and other organizations currently are in the business of supporting quality management systems within the managed care industry. Some rely on clinical databases, while others use claims or other information collected by the MCO from its participating providers. As yet, none of these systems are comprehensive in scope, focusing, as they do, primarily on hospital-based activity and thereby failing to capture sufficient ambulatory care data. It is likely that these systems will be substantially improved as they evolve. Therefore, it is important that both MCOs and their participating physicians be committed to applying this new technology if it is ever to realize its promise.

Provision of high quality health services has become such a critical basic issue in the managed care industry that MCOs are realizing that they will need to commit substantial resources to measuring and managing quality. Despite society's loud and clear concern about the cost of health care, an equally loud and clear message is being sent calling for quality maintenance and improvements. The call represents a significant challenge to physicians, managed care organizations, and to the whole health care industry, as well.

Most experts in the managed care field will readily concede that there may indeed be individual MCOs that provide inferior care, just as there are isolated incidents of inferior care provided in the non-managed care sector. But various studies suggest that the quality of care provided within managed care arrangements overall is at least equal, or perhaps even slightly superior, to that which is available in the community in which they are located. The Group Health Association of America in April 1991 distributed a fact sheet listing some interesting relevant findings. Here are some excerpts from that fact sheet:

> *In its 12-year, $80 million health insurance experiment, RAND Corporation concluded that regardless of enrollees' income levels or health status, "the cost savings achieved... through lower hospitalization rates were not reflected in lower levels of health status." (Annuals of Internal Medicine, January 5, 1987)*

> *A study of the quality of ambulatory care received for 17 chronic conditions by a general population of 6,000 adults enrolled in the RAND Health Insurance Experiment found that those persons randomized to an HMO had slightly better overall quality of care than those in the fee-for-service system. (Medical Care, May 1990, Vol. 28, No. 5)*

> *Results from the National Medicare Competition Evaluation covering the demonstration phase of the Medicare risk contracting program indicate that Medicare beneficiaries in HMOs are significantly more likely than those in fee-for-service medicine to receive care that includes complete medical histories, screening examinations, and screening tests. The author of the study concludes that "the care received in an HMO is much more likely to be complete and coordinated."*

> *Ninety-three percent of HMO users in a survey of 1,500 Americans are satisfied with the quality of their physician care. Of those with fee-for-service coverage, 89 percent are either very satisfied or somewhat satisfied with their doctors' care. (Health Insurance Association of America)*

The challenge for the 1990s will be to further enhance physicians' and MCOs' ability to improve the quality of health care.

Utilization Management

Obviously, a close relationship exists between an MCO's quality management and utilization management systems. It is not surprising, therefore, that, as with terminology related to quality assurance, the term "utilization review" is now being replaced by the term "utilization management." And, as in discussions of quality, the change in utilization terminology also signals a shift in focus from a retrospective process to a more concurrent and proactive involvement.

The change in utilization terminology also signals a shift in focus from a retrospective process to a more concurrent and proactive involvement.

The relationship between utilization management and cost containment needs to be understood in the context of managed care objectives. The focus must be on managing utilization and assuring that patients and physicians are utilizing resources appropriately. The outcome of this process usually is a containment of costs realized through the reduction of unnecessary or inappropriate services. However, it should be noted that the utilization of certain health services, such as some physician office visits and certain other ambulatory services, can and should actually increase as a result of introducing managed care. It is worth noting that most of the utilization review approaches current in the industry still reflect a retrospective, rather than current or prospective approach. This fact illustrates the degree to which a commitment to upgrading utilization (and quality) management systems is needed.

Figures 18 and 19 illustrate the kinds of utilization review and other cost control measures most frequently used by HMOs. Other types of MCOs also rely on many of the same measures, provided that their structures permit them to do so.

Most studies show that effective utilization management can, in fact, improve the quality of care. The above-cited RAND study, for example, found that lower hospital utilization rates did not diminish the health status of HMO members. It further noted that "HMO members experience up to 40 percent fewer admissions and save up to 28 percent on health care costs compared to those in a fee-for-service system," and that "inpatient utilization rates in HMOs were substantially below the national average for 1988." Established HMOs provided 358 inpatient days per 1,000 enrollees under the age 65, in contrast to a national average of 519 days per 1,000, the study reported. HMO rates for those 65 and older were found to be 1,582 days per 1,000 as compared to a national average of 2,970.

> Most studies show that effective utilization management can, in fact, improve the quality of care.

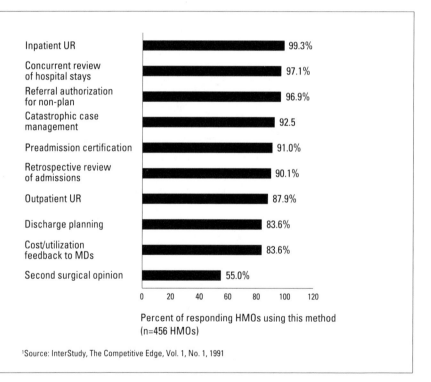

Figure 18
HMO Utilization Review (UR)[1]
Measures Used to Control Costs

Inpatient UR	99.3%
Concurrent review of hospital stays	97.1%
Referral authorization for non-plan	96.9%
Catastrophic case management	92.5
Preadmission certification	91.0%
Retrospective review of admissions	90.1%
Outpatient UR	87.9%
Discharge planning	83.6%
Cost/utilization feedback to MDs	83.6%
Second surgical opinion	55.0%

Percent of responding HMOs using this method
(n=456 HMOs)

[1]Source: InterStudy, The Competitive Edge, Vol. 1, No. 1, 1991

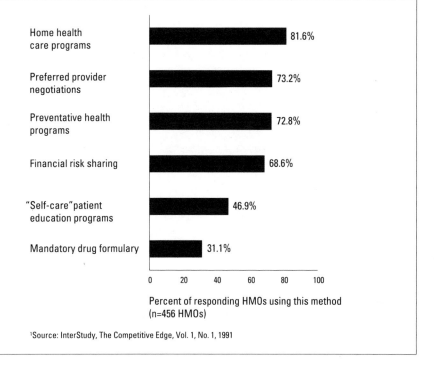

Figure 19
**Other HMO
Cost Control
Measures[1]**

Home health care programs — 81.6%

Preferred provider negotiations — 73.2%

Preventative health programs — 72.8%

Financial risk sharing — 68.6%

"Self-care" patient education programs — 46.9%

Mandatory drug formulary — 31.1%

0 20 40 60 80 100

Percent of responding HMOs using this method
(n=456 HMOs)

[1]Source: InterStudy, The Competitive Edge, Vol. 1, No. 1, 1991

Savings generated from such utilization management activities can either be passed back to the consumer through a reduced rate of premium increases, or back to providers as incentives for producing greater value in the health care system, or both.

During the 1990s, physicians will be provided with a host of new management systems technology to assist them in prospectively managing the utilization of managed care patients, including treatment profiles and protocols available in the doctor's office through electronic means. The MCOs most likely to survive the decade are already making plans to invest in this technology. Improvements in the ambulatory care component of utilization management systems also can be expected as the trend from inpatient to ambulatory services continues.

> Poorly designed and/or administered quality and utilization management systems can raise barriers to necessary care and thereby eventually increase cost and reduce quality.

Poorly designed and/or administered quality and utilization management systems can, of course, have exactly the opposite effect than they are intended to have, raising barriers to necessary care and thereby eventually increasing cost and reducing quality. Although this has been known to happen, most MCOs have recognized this potential threat and either already have or are in the process of rehabilitating their approaches to quality and utilization management. Those that are unwilling or incapable of doing so can only expect to become the casualties of the current decade.

The Hassle Factor

A final consideration to weigh in assessing an MCO's support systems is what might be called "the hassle factor." Inordinate paperwork requirements, clumsy referral authorization and preadmission certifications systems, and the like are not unknown to MCOs. Fortunately, as organizations mature, processes like these tend to become more streamlined. As automated support systems and objective evaluation techniques develop, they tend to help MCOs identify which physicians need to be closely monitored and which do not. Once that capability is in place, MCOs are likely to relax procedures for physicians who routinely meet established standards. It benefits both parties, then, when physicians and MCOs work together to design systems and procedures that contribute to the minimalization of the hassle factor.

Sizing up an MCO

Any physician considering entering into an association with an MCO should evaluate the MCO as carefully as the MCO evaluates physicians. Recognizing the many kinds of MCOs that exist and the wide variations among them, it is essential to determine how any one MCO is likely to represent the proper fit between the physician's own objectives, preferences, and style.

An exhaustive analytical evaluation of any MCO may not be possible without the advice of an expert in MCO analysis, an approach that is likely to be prohibitively costly for any single physician, or even for a small group of physicians. There are, however, less costly ways in which to accomplish at least part of this analysis.

Few better sources of information on an MCO exist than the physicians who are actually participating in it. A casual lunch or dinner discussion, focused around the issues illuminated by this book and the checklist provided in it, could elicit a great deal of information. Rather than relying on any one subjective evaluation, however, an even better idea may be to supplement individual interviews with a structured discussion that brings several physicians participating in the MCO together with several of your colleagues who share your interest in it. These strategies represent relatively easy, inexpensive ways to sort out what MCOs actually do from what they say they will do.

> Few better sources of information on an MCO exist than the physicians who are actually participating in it.

State and federal regulatory authorities are other good sources of information. State regulatory agencies, most typically departments of insurance and/or public health, require HMOs to submit reports that can be helpful in determining their financial status and growth patterns. Few states, however, regulate PPOs; therefore, reports of their activities may not be available. It also may be possible to determine if member or provider complaints about an MCO have been filed with these agencies, or if the agency has placed an MCO on an alert status because of an unsound financial situation.

Information filed with regulatory agencies will, of course, be in the form of financial and gross utilization statistics and will not deal with many of the specific issues that may be on a physician's mind. But these statistics will provide certain baseline data for use in an evaluation. Requesting reports on an annual basis will also provide the interested physician with a means for tracking an MCO's ongoing progress.

Table 11 identifies some key financial ratios that can be used to evaluate an HMO, provided that appropriate financial data is available. Although the ratios identified in Table 11 are primarily baseline indicators, they can provide some indication of an HMO's viability. In the

Table 11
HMO Financial Ratios

	Definition	Desired Range
Profitability		
Profit margin (as %)	Net income divided by revenue	>2%
Net worth (% change)	Average annual change in net worth	>1%
Capitalization		
Debt ratio (%)	Total unsubordinated debt divided by net assets	<75%
Debt service coverage ratio	Net income + depreciation and interest, divided by annual principal and interest changes	>2.0
Liquidity		
Current ratio	Current assets divided by current liabilities	>1.0
Asset test	Cash + market securities divided by current liabilities	>0.25
Premium receivable turnover	Premium receivables divided by premium revenue per month	<0.25
Cash to claims and payables	Cash + market securities + premium receivables, divided by total unpaid claims + accounts payable	>1.0
Average claims payment period	Claims payable divided by total medical cost per month (including hospital expense)	<1.0
Inpatient IBNR payment period	Inpatient IBNR divided by inpatient expense per month	<2.0
Physician IBNR payment period	Physician IBNR divided by physician expense per month	<2.0
Referral IBNR payment period	Referral IBNR divided by referral expense per month	<2.0
Other medical IBNR payment period	Other medical IBNR divided by other medical expense per month	<2.0
Total IBNR payment period	Total IBNR divided by total related expenses per month	<2.0
IBNR as percentage of claims	Total IBNR divided by total unpaid claims	<50%
Claims as percentage of revenue	Total unpaid claims divided by revenue	<15%
Efficiency		
Medical loss ratio*(%) (aka health care delivery expense)	Total medical costs (incl. hospital) divided by revenue	<85%
Administrative cost ratio (%)	Total administrative expenses divided by revenue	<15%
Medical loss PMPM**	Total medical costs divided by member months (aka health care delivery expense PMPM)	***
Premium revenue PMPM	Premium revenue divided by member months	***
Physician expense PMPM	Physician expenses divided by member months	***
Hospital expense PMPM	Hospital expenses divided by member months	***
Other professional expense PMPM	Other professional expenses divided by member months	***
Other medical expense PMPM	Other medical expenses divided by member months	***
Net income PMPM	Net income divided by member months	***
% growth in premium PMPM	Average annual change in premium per member month	>1 %
% growth in member months	Average annual change in member months	>1 %
Composition		
Receivables to current assets (%)	Premium receivables divided by current assets	<75%
Cash to current assets (%)	Cash + market securities divided by current assets	>25%

*Medical loss ratio is a term used by state departments of insurance and HMO market analysis.

**PMPM = per member per month.

***These figures are dependent on the plan's age and model type; therefore, no recommended range is given.

Source: Healthcare Data Bank, Sebastapol, CA

case of regulated companies, the financial data needed to determine these ratios should be available from the appropriate state regulatory agency. In many states, MCO regulation is the responsibility of the insurance or health department, or the state department of corporations. In some states, however, regulatory authority is shared by two departments. In the case of companies that are not regulated, relevant data would have to be obtained directly from the MCO itself. It should also be noted that interpreting this information may require the expertise of an independent advisor.

"How to Check Out an HMO," an article originally published in the June 1989 *Business Week* and reprinted here as Appendix D, also can suggest some questions that might be raised in evaluating an MCO. Although specifically addressed to employers, the information it provides should also be useful to potential providers.

Statistical data will not, of course, tell physicians everything they may need or want to know about an MCO. Many other factors need to be considered in identifying predictors of success or failure. The vision and leadership skills of an MCO's board members, management, and physician leaders may be at least as important to its future as its financial performance to date.

We can also learn from history at least where some of the major pitfalls for MCOs may lie. Table 12, which summarizes almost 30 years of MCO analysis and observations by the author, lists the most common reasons for MCO failures. Reviewed together with the criteria for success outlined in Appendix E, it should offer a good road map to the decision-making process.

Table 12
Common Reasons for Managed Care Organization Failures

- Ineffective board and management leadership
- Undercapitalization and underresourcing of key functions
- Inadequate management controls and management information systems
- Failure to develop effective quality management systems
- Poorly designed health care delivery systems (networks)
- Failure to effectively *manage* health care costs (unit costs and frequency)
- Ineffective or counterproductive provider incentive system design
- Ineffective claims management and faulty claims accounting and accruing
- Poorly defined and managed underwriting and premium setting
- Obsolete products, provider support systems, member support systems, etc.
- Failure to develop and execute effective strategic business planning processes

Chapter 4:

Planning for the Future

Forecasting the future is a risky business in any area of

endeavor, and no less so in managed care. In the 1980s, for

example, conventional wisdom had it that the managed care

business would be dominated by a small number of "super-

meds" by the 1990s. The prediction never came true, and for

reasons that should always have been apparent: managed care

is a *local* business that depends on *local* physicians and what occurs at the doctor-patient interface. The physician's relationship with the rest of the delivery system is also a local variable. Such relationships must be developed and fostered at the local level and can be neither legislated nor managed from distant centralized headquarters.

Despite the cost to some of this major forecasting miscalculation, the need to prepare for the future by trying to anticipate what it may hold remains. And the better we understand what has happened in the past, the better able we should be to determine what may occur in the future.

The significant geographical variations that have been experienced throughout the country with regard to the acceptance of managed care offer special opportunities for 20/20 foresight to those in areas where that acceptance has lagged. Experience indicates that certain market dynamics are inevitable as markets mature. Those in areas where managed care has not yet become well established have much to learn from the experience of those in more mature markets.

For example, it appears to be safe to assume that growth in managed care in nonmetropolitan and rural areas will continue to lag behind growth in urban areas. However, a number of successful rural HMOs currently do operate in the US, suggesting that some rural areas can anticipate a steady increase in managed care activity during the coming decade. Allowances must be made, of course, for variables such as local economics, geographical barriers, and other factors. However, understanding the growth strategies of existing MCOs makes it clear why greater penetration into rural areas is inevitable.

> Most health care reform proposals rely heavily on managed care as a cornerstone of reform.

As metropolitan markets become saturated, MCOs typically target what they call "secondary markets" as their next area for potential growth. These secondary markets are frequently geographically adjacent markets that fall just beyond the immediate metropolitan market where the MCO initiated its business. Once the secondary market has been penetrated, MCOs usually expand to a third-tier market, which sometimes includes rural areas. Therefore, depending upon the current level of managed care market saturation within a given market, the likelihood of an MCO expanding into adjacent markets can be determined.

One common misunderstanding that may cloud forecasts of the future is an assumption that passage of some form of national health insurance or health care reform will signal the end of managed care in this country. Quite the opposite is likely to occur. Unless the nation is to be bankrupted by the cost of health care, any health care financing program will inevitably have to be coupled with a means of delivering more cost-effective health care services. Since that has been exactly the capability that good MCOs have been developing, most current health care reform proposals rely heavily on managed care as a cornerstone of reform.

Eleven Likely Trends

A trend is, by definition, a general direction or movement. In other words, although it describes an ongoing process, it will not necessary have exactly the same impact on everything or everyone in its wake at exactly the same time.

It is important to keep that fact in mind in reading the following discussion of trends in managed care. Of necessity, the trends we will be reviewing are national in scope. Exactly how, when, and even whether they may affect each individual physician will depend upon variables present in the physician's local situation. Current health system reform proposals favored by government health policy makers would convert much of the entire health care system to managed care.

1. Continued Steady Growth of Managed Care Market Share

In view of the volatility of the health care industry, projecting growth in any one segment of it is a high-risk venture indeed. Nonetheless, many experts predict that 70-80 percent or more of the US population may be receiving their health care through some type of managed care product by the turn of the century even without major reform initiatives. Several other trends support the assumptions underlying their projections.

InterStudy, the managed care research organization based in Minneapolis, has identified five managed care trends that can be anticipated for the 1990s:

- Unrestricted indemnity insurance is being phased out and will probably represent no more than 5-10 percent of the market within the next five to 10 years.
- The focus of managed care will shift even more closely to controlling the cost of care.
- Consumers will have less choice of providers.
- Providers will have less independence in making choices regarding care.
- There will be a movement away from defined benefits plans to defined contribution plans.

While the first four of these trends should be self-explanatory, the last may warrant some explanation. It refers to an effort on the part of the insurance industry to encourage greater cost-sharing on the part of employees covered by employer-sponsored plans.

Under a defined benefit plan, an employer pays the full amount to provide its employees' health benefits. Under a defined contribution plan, an employer contributes a fixed amount but offers a selection of health plans to employees, some of which cost more than others, but also may offer more to beneficiaries. The employee is free to select the more costly coverage, but must pay the difference between the defined contribution and the cost of the coverage. Thus, if an employee chose to select a more costly health benefits plan, he or she would pay more out of pocket for health care than if a less costly option were selected. The intent, of course, is to encourage employees to become more aware of the best values-for-dollar among their options and, as a result, evaluate their options from the perspective of a prudent buyer.

A blurring of the distinctions between HMOs, PPOs, and other managed care products is expected to continue and accelerate in the coming years. PPOs already are beginning to look more and more like HMOs in terms of the degree of influence they have over the delivery of care, and, as markets mature, there is likely to be movement away from such transition products and toward more tightly structured products. It is likely that Medicare and Medicaid beneficiaries will be required to receive their care through some form of managed care.

2. An Acute Shortage of Primary Care Physicians and a Surplus in Certain Subspecialties

Many managed care products incorporate the patient manager or "gatekeeper" concept, which requires the patient to access the primary care physician prior to seeking subspecialty or other care, except in chronic cases. As a result, the demand for primary care physicians per 1,000 population for such a managed care product is higher than it is in the non-managed care arena. Therefore, the growth of the managed care industry will further intensify the already acute shortage (in some markets) of primary care physicians.

Indeed, the demand for primary care physicians per 1,000 population may more than double in an area when managed care market share goes from 0 to 50 percent or more. While this demand will probably encourage the shift of a larger percentage of the health care dollar toward the purchase of certain cognitive skills that are essential to effective patient management, the good news for primary care physicians cannot be delivered without a qualifier. Most MCOs are already developing databases that eventually will permit them to objectively evaluate provider performance. Those who do not develop the skills required to practice effective, high-quality primary care can expect the demand to pass them by.

> But at the very least, all subspecialists must learn how to measure and prove the value of their services.

Nor are prospects bright for many subspecialists. As a result, it is realistic to anticipate a significant surplus of some subspecialists as the demand for their services per 1,000 population is eroded by managed care market share growth and other factors at play in today's health care system. Some subspecialists might respond by changing their practice specialty to primary care. But at the very least, all subspecialists must learn how to measure and prove the value of their services.

3. An Increased Demand for Greater Value from the Health Care Dollar

At one time, doctors' and hospitals' assertions that they were high quality health care providers were accepted as statements of fact. During the 1980s, however, scrutiny of the cost and quality of care became intense as major health care purchasers began looking for more than anecdotal proof of these assurances. Today, there is a clear imperative for objective standards to be applied in measuring and managing the effectiveness of health care services as prudent buyers of these expensive services demand value for their dollars.

As is true of the purchasers of all kinds of products and services, the purchasers of health care define value as a function of three factors: quality, service, and cost. The higher the cost, the lower the value. The higher the quality and service, the higher the value.

Lacking substantive change in the health care system, payers interested in containing costs have had little choice but to simply discount fees and/or reduce benefits. But discounting alone is an inherently dysfunctional approach since it simply provides incentives for the provision of more services by providers. Neither discounting nor benefits reduction can, in the long-term, serve the interests of patients, providers, or the major health care purchasers.

As the major purchasers of health care struggle to define and measure quality, physicians and other providers must either take the lead in that effort or watch others take the job away from them. That means that providers must become well versed in technology now being developed to measure and monitor the cost and quality of care. If the health care professions do not take leadership positions in this arena now, it is not unlikely that they will find themselves subject to standards and monitoring techniques designed by others.

In finding ways to measure quality and the appropriateness of costs, health care providers should not lose sight of the fact that purchasers no longer are willing to evaluate the cost of care based primarily on the cost of a particular service, such as a single office visit or hospital day. Rather, they now are viewing costs in terms of the total cost of all health care services per person per year. This much more comprehensive focus in turn demands a much more comprehensive approach to managing the cost of all of the care an individual may receive during a given year.

Managed care has afforded some success in achieving this objective. Although it is by no means either a panacea or the only way in which to produce greater value in health care, it does offer an organized and systematic approach to solving the problem that would never be possible if it were sought on the basis of one physician or one hospital at a time. Various other approaches will undoubtedly be identified as the struggle to maximize value continues. By the turn of the century, the term managed care, as we now know it, may itself have become obsolete. Nonetheless, it is safe to assume that, whatever approaches are finally devised, whatever they come to be called, they will inevitably be built on what has been learned and is still being learned as the managed care industry takes shape.

4. Intensification of the Shift in Focus from Inpatient to Ambulatory Care Management

During the 1980s, most successful MCOs were able to reduce levels of hospital utilization from 800-900 days of care per 1,000 population to 300-400 days per 1,000, and some are now targeting further reductions to as low as 100 days or less by the end of the decade. That task was relatively easy to manage because of the relatively few occasions of care (that is, admissions to the hospital) and relatively few sites of care (just one or only a few hospitals) that were involved in the achievement of their mission.

Now, however, the focus is rapidly shifting to the ambulatory care portion of the health care delivery system as pressure builds to control costs in that segment of the health care industry. That challenge will not be so easily met, given the many more and varied sites at which ambulatory care may be provided and the far greater number of individual services involved. It is likely that an entirely new level of management technology will be required to success-fully achieve this goal, much of it involving clinical databases and automated clinical decision-making support systems. Physicians should be taking the lead in the development of this technology.

5. A Continued Shift in Underwriting Risk from Insurers to Providers

Prior to managed care, providers were reimbursed on a fee-for-service or cost-plus basis. Employers and insurers assumed all of the risk for the care their employers and beneficiaries would need. Managed care tends to shift this underwriting risk to providers, particularly if capitation is the method of payment used by payers. It is expected that capitation may become the most prevalent form of provider payment during this decade.

As risk is shifted from one component of the insurance marketplace to another, the organization or provider to which the risk is shifted must, of course, be capable of successfully managing that risk. This will require certain tools, most importantly, reporting mechanisms to provide essential information, including information that will permit comparisons of actual performance by individual physicians against established standards. Other essential tools will include provider incentive systems, and utilization and quality management systems.

MCOs that are committed to their own long-term success must be equally committed to making their providers successful, providing them with these essential tools. Physicians, on their part, can demonstrate to patients and purchasers of care their dedication to increasing the value of services rendered by learning how to use these tools effectively.

6. Intense Competition Among and Continued Consolidation of MCOs

Since 1987, when the number of HMOs in the US reached its peak, 25 to 50 HMOs have either been acquired by or merged with another HMO or gone out of business almost every year. The decline in numbers of HMOs is expected to continue throughout the 1990s, and a similar trend can be expected among PPOs as enrollment continues to increase. However, total HMO enrollment has continued to increase. Both HMOs and PPOs, which historically have focused on single markets and single products, now are expanding into adjacent markets in an ongoing effort to increase enrollment. Regionalization is well underway.

> The decline in numbers of HMOs is expected to continue throughout the 1990s, and a similar trend can be expected among PPOs as enrollment continues to increase.

The decline in numbers of MCOs is being fueled by several other factors, as well, among them, an increasing desire on the part of employers to reduce the number of insurance-type contracts they must administer. The long-term objective for many employers is to contract with just one company that can offer a full spectrum of managed care and other insurance products.

As a means toward that end, some employers, such as the State of California, have established criteria that must be met by MCOs that wish to continue contracting with them. Typically, these criteria require the MCO to have in place a health care delivery system or network that is sufficiently broadly-based geographically to enable it to serve employees wherever they live. Some employers also are establishing minimum enrollment levels below which enrollment in an MCO may not fall if it wishes to continue to contract with the employer.

Some small but increasingly significant economies of scale can be realized when MCOs obtain certain enrollment levels. For example, administrative costs of an HMO with 30,000-50,000 members might represent as much as 15 percent or more of total premium revenues. In contrast, administrative costs of an HMO with 200,000-300,000 members might be as low as 8 or 9 percent, and the figure in those with enrollments of a million may be as low as 5 or 6 percent.

However, to the physician concerned with affiliating with organizations that promise the greatest likelihood of success, an HMO's size is not necessarily the best indicator. Some of the biggest MCOs that have entered the managed care business to date have produced some of the biggest failures. Conversely, some smaller local and regional companies are operating quite effectively and may enjoy considerable success in the future. In the last analysis, each MCO must be evaluated on its own merit.

7. Managed Care Product Line Diversification

The managed care product line spectrum illustrated by Figure 1, which appears on page 9, suggests that relatively clear distinctions exist between HMOs, PPOs, and the rest of the health insurance market. That certainly was the case in the 1970s and in the early 1980s, when most MCOs were still single-product companies. As we have seen, however, a number of factors are now driving MCOs toward product diversification and blending in the interest of enabling individuals to select among a variety of offerings, all of them available through one managed care organization. Meanwhile, so-called "point-of-service" plans are producing hybrid versions of managed care products that further blur distinctions.

The trend promises to leave physicians who are affiliated with single-product MCOs vulnerable as market demand for more comprehensive products rises. Physicians concerned about the future therefore would be well advised to seek assurances that any MCOs with which they contract plan to and have the ability to move beyond traditional single product lines.

8. Continued Blending of Delivery System Models

As we have seen, distinctions between staff model, group practice model, IPA model, network model, and direct contracting model MCOs are rapidly disappearing, as are distinctions between managed care products. Managed care organizations that historically have been adamant about maintaining the "purity" of the model on which they are based now are recognizing the need for expanding their provider base in order to respond to market demands. Thus, organizations such as the Kaiser and Prudential health plans, which have historically been based on group practice models, are now exploring the IPA model. It can be anticipated that this blending of models will continue during the 1990s, albeit with continuing movement toward the right side of the product line spectrum, as depicted in Figure 1.

This movement represents a natural evolution as MCOs compete with each other for market share by developing more effective cost and quality management systems. The trend also may represent increased opportunity for physicians to participate on an individual basis with MCOs that historically have operated only through a closed-panel structure.

9. Declining Differences Between Managed Care and Indemnity Utilization Patterns

When the managed care industry was in its infancy in the early 1970s, the typical non-managed care population under the age of 65 utilized hospital days at a rate of 800-900 days per 1,000. At that time, it was relatively easy for an MCO to enter the market and almost immediately reduce that rate to 500-600 days per 1,000, and to realize further reductions to 300-400 days over time. In the last 10 to 15 years, during which most physicians in metropolitan areas have participated in at least one MCO, the patient management skills they have learned from managed care have also been applied more broadly to the management of all their patients. Obviously realizing the benefits of this change in practice patterns, the utilization rates of indemnity insurance plan beneficiaries have now begun to follow the same pattern as those experienced by MCOs.

> Utilization rates of indemnity insurance plans have now begun to follow the same pattern as those experienced by MCOs.

A similar phenomenon has been documented within smaller environments, such as group practices that are serving both fee-for-service and managed care patients. As physicians within the group adopt new styles and standards of practice, they tend to apply them to all patients, with less and less regard for whether or not the care of an individual patient is paid for by a managed care organization.

It is unlikely that indemnity insurance plans will ever attain the same level of efficiency as tightly-structured MCOs, nor is it likely that the presence of MCOs is the only reason for the declining hospital utilization trend. But this shift in utilization patterns does suggest the value to all when providers learn new practice styles. The utilization trend further suggests that MCOs will need to continue to improve their methodologies and management technologies if they are to retain their competitive edge.

10. Increased Capital Demands to Pay for Development of New Management and Systems Technology

The managed care industry is only beginning to emerge from its adolescence, and thus now stands on the brink of substantial refinement of some of the basics of its business. Where once both business management and clinical management technology were lacking in the industry, considerable effort and capital is now being invested in development of this technology, which will become a standard component of most successful MCOs before the end of the decade. These new systems will make it possible to identify the level of physician performance. Thus, successful MCOs of the future will have the ability to identify providers who demonstrate superior performance, and to reward them accordingly, while taking appropriate steps to deal with those who do not meet established standards.

11. Continued Pressure on Health Care Costs as the Result of Normal Economic Cycles

As Figure 19 illustrates, the pattern of underwriting cycles that have occurred among Blue Cross/Blue Shield plans during a period of 25 consecutive years is one of three years of gain followed by three years of loss. The pattern is common to the entire health insurance industry, including the managed care segment. It is important to understand this cycle in order to place in perspective MCO financial trends.

During the last two years of the 1980s, for example, MCOs' financial performance was extremely poor. Some critics tended to conclude from that fact that the managed care industry was faltering, failing to recognize that the performance of the managed care segment of the health insurance industry was only part of a larger industry cycle.

The fact that these cycles occur, however, does not mean that physicians need not be concerned with the financial strength of an MCO they may be considering. In fact, as Figure 19 further illustrates, the downturns have been deeper with each cycle, a fact that suggests that organizations that fail to get control over the cost of care will be extremely vulnerable during the down cycles of the 1990s. In fact, it will probably become increasingly difficult for marginal MCOs to survive these cycles, while those that take appropriate steps to enhance their value to consumers and support their providers in the provision of high-quality, cost-effective care should be in a better position to build the reserves they need to survive natural gain/loss cycles.

A Final Word

As we have seen, change in the US health care system appears inevitable. It is an inevitability that physicians can view either as a threat or an opportunity. It is hoped that the information presented in this book will help physicians understand how they may create those opportunities as they continue to improve the health care provided their patients. Certainly the knowledge that they can do so should help allay some of the anxieties physicians may experience as they anticipate the future.

However, information alone is not enough to assure physicians a secure future. Action is needed, and it must be guided by a carefully crafted and implemented action plan.

The key to developing an action plan is to focus on appropriate objectives and to understand the environment well enough to make realistic clinical, strategic, business, and personal decisions. Understanding the concepts underlying managed care and the need to maximize value at the point of doctor-patient interface is an essential first step. So, too, is understanding whether, when, and how to organize to assure the maximization of value. It has been said before, but it warrants repeating: organizing simply to preserve the status quo is only likely to place physicians in an even more vulnerable position as society continues to sound its demands for change.

Change is opportunity, and the time to take charge of it is now.

Appendix A — Questions for Physicians Who Are Considering Managed Care Options

This list is oriented around primary care physicians, but many of the questions are applicable to subspecialists as well.

1. *Breadth of clinical abilities.* What services will I be expected and allowed to provide without referral? Will I be able to practice the breadth of my practice? Am I responsible for all health care costs the patient incurs, or only those defined as the "primary care" costs? Am I in full control of those "primary care costs"?

   Typical clinical responsibilities for primary care physicians participating in a managed health care program may include:

   - care for patients of all ages — neonatal through geriatric
   - provide preventive counseling, testing, and other services
   - provide health maintenance procedures, routine health care for all ages (history, examinations, screening procedures, immunizations, anticipatory guidance, risk identification and reduction, etc)
   - perform office procedures (eg, sigmoidoscopy, vasectomy, lump and bump removal, endometrial biopsy, etc)
   - provide basic mental health services/counseling
   - provide health education services
   - provide care in all settings: hospital, home, extended care, and nursing facilities
   - arrange for appropriate referral to other health care professionals
   - coordinate care across providers and settings
   - provide accessibility to primary care services 24 hours/day, seven days/week, including telephone consultation and follow-up
   - provide prenatal, labor and delivery, postpartum care — consistent with training and experience (special issues — see 3 below)

2. *Ability to function as the case manager.* Do I retain the role of provider of all care and make all decisions about consultation/referral when necessary? Are patients required to seek my approval before other providers can be accessed? Do I receive reports from all providers and maintain a complete record of the patient's health care? Who are the consultants available to me? Do I have confidence in their ability and interactive skills? How much control do I have in the decision of when, where, and to whom to refer my patients? Am I reimbursed for the complexities of the case management role?

3. *Obstetrics.* Am I able/willing to provide complete obstetric care? If so, will the plan allow me to do so? Will it pay me to do so? If not providing intrapartum care, will I be able to provide prenatal care? Who will be my back-up for complications? What will my role be intrapartum? Postpartum? If I do not provide any obstetric care, what are the procedures for referral to another specialist? Will the patient continue to see me during and after the pregnancy for other problems? Does the plan consider obstetrician/gynecologists to be primary care physicians? Will I be able to provide care for the newborn?

4. *Principles of cost-effective health care and clinical decision-making.* Am I confident in my ability to perform a wide scope of primary care services in a cost-effective manner? Do the cost-containment requirements of the HMO compromise my clinical decision-making in any way which adversely affects patients? If so, what mechanisms are there to ensure that a balance between physician and autonomy, cost-containment, and quality of care is achieved?

5. *Reimbursement for physician services.* Does the managed care entity provide equivalent payment for all primary care physicians who provide the same services, regardless of specialty? Whom does the HMO consider to be "primary care" physicians?

Additional Questions

- Are you and your staff prepared to accept financial risks for the cost of care?
- Are you prepared to *manage* patients? (It means saying *no* from time to time.)
- Will your office structure (furniture/exam rooms) withstand any patient volume increases?
- Will your medical records withstand detailed scrutiny?
- Will your bookkeeping/accounting system be able to track accruals?
- Will you be able to track patients — new, concurrent, and those who lose their coverage?
- Are you prepared to provide and document mandated benefits:
  – EPSDT
  – Screening exams
  – Education services
- Are you prepared to collect co-payments and coordination of benefits revenue?
- Do you share calls with another contractor physician?
- Could your office pass inspection for fire code violations by a fire marshall?
- Do you thoroughly understand the nature of your risks, and are you prepared to manage that risk?

Adapted from Eidus, Robert, MD, and Samuel W. Warburton, MD. *Managed Care: A Teaching Syllabus,* Society of Teachers of Family Medicine, Kansas City, MO. May 1990.

Appendix B   Non-Covered Services (Example)

- Out-of-Area Non-Emergency Services
- Medical and Ancillary Services
- Care for military service-connected disability for which *member* is legally entitled to services and for which facilities are reasonably available to this *member*. Care for conditions that state or local laws require to be treated in a public facility.
- Custodial, Domiciliary Care, or Rest Cures.
- Cosmetic Surgery, unless medically indicated.
- Experimental medical, surgical, or other experimental health care procedures unless approved as a basic health care service by the MCO policy-making body, and considered non-experimental by the national medical community at large.
- Except in event of Emergency Hospital services, the *member* shall not be entitled to hospital benefits hereunder unless such confinement is at the direction of any attending participating physician.
- Personal Comfort Items.
- Sex Change Operations and Reversal of Voluntarily Induced Infertility.
- In Vitro Fertilization.
- The cost of care for bodily injury or sickness arising out of or in the course of the *member's* employment, which is compensable under any Worker's Compensation or Occupational Disease Act or Law. Provider shall coordinate benefits with the appropriate carrier(s) for reimbursement.

Adapted from Warburton, Samuel W., MD, *Evaluating Prepaid Contracts.* Annual Workshop for Directors of Family Residency Programs, June 6 and 7, 1988.

Appendix C — Primary Care Physician Services (Example)

1. Services of primary care physicians and other health professionals and supplies provided in physician's office. These services include routine office visits, minor office surgical procedures, immunizations, injections, periodic physical examinations, and other usual and customary care.

2. Primary care physician visits and examinations, including consultation time and treatment, telephone consultations, and time for personal attendance with the member during a confinement in a hospital, skilled nursing facility, or other covered facility.

3. Physician services in member's home when the nature of the member's illness indicates.

4. Well-child care from birth (excluding the initial newborn hospital visit by physician).

5. Periodic health appraisal evaluations (including all periodic examinations recommended under the appropriate health maintenance standards adopted by HMO).

6. Pediatric and adult immunizations in accordance with the recommendations of the American Academy of Pediatrics, the Federal Centers for Disease Control, HMO's policies, and other appropriate agencies and professional societies. Capitation rates or compensation will be adjusted as determined by HMO to reflect significant changes in either the cost of vaccines or the schedule of immunizations.

7. Vision and hearing screening of members through 17 years of age (excluding refractions for vision corrective prescriptions).

8. Family planning services as set forth in applicable certificates of coverage.

9. Medical care services available seven days per week, 24 hours per day.

10. Laboratory procedures routinely performed in a primary care physician's office, including urinalysis, vaginal wet drop, throat cultures, tuberculin test, drawing blood, and specimen collection.

11. Education services to (a) assist members to make appropriate use of health care services; (b) provide information to members about personal health behavior; and (c) provide information to members about achieving and maintaining physical and mental health.

Note: These services listed represent typical primary care services under primary care capitation arrangements. Actual definitions of primary care services depend on the specific HMO and community.

Adapted from Wagner, Eric R., Principal. *A Practical Guide to Evaluating Physician Capitation Payments.* The American Society of Internal Medicine, Publication Number 337 (2.5M:7/87), 1987.

Appendix D — "How to Check Out an HMO"

Before you sign that HMO contract, you might want to get answers to the items on this checklist.

The key to a solid relationship between you and an HMO is understanding in advance what you're buying. That means knowing more about the product than simply how much you're going to pay every month.

What follows is a checklist of important questions and items you might want to answer or verify before contracting with an HMO. The health plan should give you most of this information, however, your state's insurance and health departments and the federal Office of Prepaid Health Care under the US Health Care Financing Administration can assist you as well.

Model:

- Group
- Staff
- Individual practice association
- Network
- Other

Ownership:

- Private, or publicly traded national holding company or HMO chain
- Commercial insurance company
- Blue Cross/Blue Shield
- Physician group
- Hospital
- Independent
- Cooperative
- Other, such as state medical assistance agency.

Licensure and qualification:

- Is the HMO federally qualified?
- Does the plan comply with federal qualification requirements ?
- Is the plan licensed by the appropriate regulatory agencies in your state, eg, health or health or insurance department?
- Is the HMO in compliance with the various financial, management and medical practice requirements of your state?
- Does the plan have a history of non-compliance with state or federal regulatory agencies?
- Are there any restrictions or pending reviews by state or federal regulatory agencies?
- Has the HMO been the defendant in any civil or criminal litigation? If so, what was the outcome? Was any employer named in these suits?
- Has the HMO been accredited by any other organization such as the Joint Commission for the Accreditation of Health Care Organizations or the American Association of Ambulatory Health Centers?

Size:

- How many contracts does the HMO have? How many of these are individual contracts? Individual plus spouse? Individual plus dependents? Medicare?
- What's been the HMO's annual growth rate?
- What are its five-year growth projections?
- What is the ratio of enrollees to physicians?
- What other employers does the HMO serve?
- Can the HMO demonstrate that it is capable of handling your group?

Benefits:

- What basic benefits does the plan offer?
- Does the HMO offer "preventive" care such as smoking cessation classes, stress management, cancer screening, etc?
- Does the HMO offer flexible benefit packages enabling enrollees to obtain medical services from non-affiliated doctors? How much does this service cost the company and the employee?
- Does the plan offer optional benefits like dental or eye-care coverage, pharmacy discounts, coverage for chiropractic care or physical therapy, home health, private-duty nurses or extended skilled nursing-facility coverage? What other supplemental benefits does the HMO offer?
- How much does each supplemental benefit cost?
- Are there limitations on mental health and psychiatric benefits and on those covering chronic illnesses such as diabetes or AIDS?
- What is the HMO's policy on experimental or catastrophic procedures such as organ transplants?
- Will members have around-the-clock access to a physician's care?
- Under what conditions may enrollees change physicians? What procedures must they follow to make the change?
- What is the HMO's policy on out-of-area coverage? How does it define an out-of-area emergency? What are the procedures for obtaining out-of-service? How are claims filed?
- Is the plan open to retirees, surviving spouses, sponsored dependents, or Medicare beneficiaries? Do benefits differ for these individuals?
- Will the HMO administer COBRA and bill beneficiaries?

Rating and data:

- What has the HMO's community rate been over the past five years?
- How will your group be rated?
- Experience: Rates are determined by actual cost of delivering medical care to your employees.
- Community rating: Rates are based on averages for the entire HMO enrollment.
- Community rating by class: Employees are classified according to some factor, like age, sex, or residence, and a rate is calculated for each group.

- Have the HMO demonstrate how it will calculate your rates for individuals, individuals plus spouse, and individuals plus family. Have rates calculated for two years. Will the plan guarantee these rates or set limits on annual increases?

- Is the plan willing to adjust its benefit package to better suit your needs and reduce premiums?

- Does the plan require any copayments or deductibles? For which benefits? Will it institute copayments or deductibles to reduce premiums?

- Can the HMO provide you with group-specific utilization data? If not, when will it have the capability to provide you with this information?

- How, if applicable, will the HMO coordinate benefits with other insurance coverage?

Marketing and service area:

- Does the plan provide all enrollees with comprehensive information about:
  - basic and supplemental benefits;
  - procedures for selecting a physician or clinic and hospital;
  - procedures for obtaining referrals;
  - procedures for arranging routine and emergency care?

- How does the HMO intend to market itself to your employees? Ask for copies of all marketing materials including brochures, posters, advertisements, meeting materials, etc.

- How many physicians does the HMO contract with? How do the locations of medical offices mesh with the geographic dispersion of your work force?

- How many primary-care physicians are available for new members and where are their offices located?

- What hospitals does the HMO contract with? Where are these hospitals in relation to where most of your employees live?

- Does the HMO's market overlap areas already served by other health plans you're contracting with? If so, would contracting with the HMO prove more cost effective than your existing arrangements?

Contractual relationships:

- Do the contracts between the HMO and its providers contain any provisions that would jeopardize the relationship between your employees and their physicians or hospitals? For example, some HMOs allow providers to cancel their contracts if after 60 days they're not satisfied with the arrangements.

- What, if any, "hold harmless" arrangements does the plan have with providers? In other words, in the event of its insolvency, does the plan guarantee that its providers will not seek payment from enrollees or their employers?

Physicians:

- By what criteria does the HMO select its primary-care physicians and its specialists?
- Are physicians employees or contractors of the HMO?
- Will the HMO allow prospective enrollees to review physician credentials?
- Is board certification required? How many physicians are certified? How many are eligible?
- By what criteria are physician contracts renewed?
- How are primary-care physicians paid? Salary? Fee-for-service? Capitation?
- If physicians are capitated, do the fees cover the cost of of office visits? Specialist referrals? Lab tests? Other?
- When do primary-care physicians receive bonuses? Are incentives based on individual or group performance?
- Under what conditions are physicians penalized for their utilization of medical services?
- Does the HMO require all physicians to carry malpractice liability insurance?

Hospitals:

- By what criteria are contracting hospitals selected?
- Are hospitals accredited by the Joint Commission for the Accreditation of Health Care Organizations?
- Do the hospitals accept Medicare and Medicaid?
- Does the HMO regularly review the quality assurance policies and financial stability of its contracting hospitals?
- How are hospitals paid? Full charges? Discounted charges? Per diem? Capitation? Other?

Other provider's qualifications:

- What criteria are used to select other providers such as physical therapists, chiropractors, pharmacies, or nursing agencies?
- Are these providers licensed with the appropriate state agencies?
- How are these providers paid?
- Does the HMO monitor their quantity?

Management:

- Who are the key managers and what is their experience?
- What is the "chain of command"? Where does the medical director fit into it?
- Who sits on the board of directors? To what degree are enrollees and the medical staff represented?
- If the HMO is part of a national chain, how much autonomy does the local management have?

Finances:

- Is the plan non-profit or for-profit?

- Is the parent company non-profit or for-profit?

- Obtain and review financial statements for the past five years. Have profits increased or decreased? If the plan has lost money, have losses improved or worsened with each year? When does the plan expect to break even?

- Evaluate past medical-loss ratios (ratios of medical expenses to premium revenue). Have the ratios increased, decreased or held constant? Do ratios meet "acceptable" industry standards, approximately 78% to 92%?

- Evaluate past ratios of administrative expenses to premium revenues. Have the ratios increased, decreased, or held constant?

- Evaluate the balance sheet for the past five years for the following:

  – trends in net worth;

  – trends in the HMO's current ratio. Are current assets greater than long current liabilities?

  – long-term liabilities: What are the covenants governing these debts? Is the HMO of abiding by these covenants?

- If a plan is part of a national or regional corporation, what percentage of the profits go back to the parent corporation?

- What are the local plan's obligations to its parent company should the parent company go bankrupt?

- If a regional or national HMO management company manages the HMO, how much does the local plan pay for these services? What other financial arrangements exist between the HMO and the management company contract with? What is its track record?

- What type of reinsurance and insolvency protection does the HMO hold?

Quality assurance:

- Obtain if possible, result of enrollee satisfaction surveys.

- What is the HMO's annual disenrollment rate?

- What has been the HMO's physician and hospital turnover rate in the past two years? What percentage of primary-care physicians and specialists have left in the past two years? Can the HMO explain the high turn-over rates?

- Obtain a copy of the HMO's quality-assurance plan. Does it call for some or all of the following:

  – provider certification or eligibility;

  – adequate malpractice coverage and monitoring of claims filed against a provider;

  – peer review;

  – chart review;

  – incident or patient-outcome review;

- a follow-up procedure for patient grievances;

- overall data review;

- corrective action; and

- follow-up.

- Has the HMO's quality assurance plan been certified by the National Committee for Quality Assurance, the Joint Commission for the Accreditation of Health Care Organizations, or another external review organization?

- Does the QA plan examine the results of utilization review surveys to ensure that medical care was appropriate?

- Does the HMO make QA reviews a condition of granting or renewing a provider's contract?

- How often and under what conditions do providers undergo QA reviews?

- Have any complaints been filed against the HMO either with the state health and/or insurance departments or with the federal Office of Prepaid Health Care? How were they resolved?

Utilization review:

- Obtain non-Medicare statistics on inpatient days per 1,000 enrollees, hospital admissions per 1,000 enrollees, and average length of stay. How do these statistics compare with local utilization trends? How may they have been affected by age or sex distribution?

- Obtain the HMO's procedures for the following:

  - prior approval for non-emergency hospital admissions;

  - concurrent review of hospitalized enrollees;

  - retrospective reviews of hospital records to ensure that care was appropriate;

  - discharge planning to ensure patients receive appropriate follow-up care;

  - ambulatory or outpatient care review to assess the appropriateness of treatment rendered in physician's offices or clinics;

  - case management to determine if it is integrated with other utilization review techniques and how these cases are identified?

- Does the HMO make participation in the UR program a condition for granting or renewing provider contracts?

- Is the HMO's UR program capable of detecting underutilization of services by providers?

This checklist was compiled by Faith Lyman Ham from the following sources: Ford Motor Co, George C. Halvorson's *How to Cut Your Company's Health Care Costs*, the Minnesota Coalition on Health's Purchasers' *Guide to Managed Health Care*, Medical Advocacy Service's *How Do the HMOs in Your Area Stack Up?*, the New York Business Group on Health's *Employers' Guide to HMOs*, Margaret E. O'Kane, director of quality management for Group Health Association, Inc, Washington, DC, A. Foster Higgins & Co Inc, and Towers Perrin & Crosby.

Business & Health/June 1989, (p. 38-40)

Criteria for Success in the Managed Care Business

1. *Clear statement of objectives for both businesses (provider and managed care) that are stated as specifically as possible in a business plan which include:*

   A. Measurable Quality of Care and Quality of Service Objectives

   B. Geographic Markets to be Targeted During Subsequent 3-5 Years (eg, Local, Statewide, Regional, etc) and Specific Market Share Objectives for Each Business

   C. Growth Objectives (eg, Patient and Member Volumes, New Product Lines, etc) and Delineation of Potential Sources of Growth for Each Business

   D. Total Managed Care Volume Desired/Required by Owner-Providers in Order to Maintain Market Share

   E. Relationship of Owner-Providers to Other Managed Care Products and Companies

   F. Financial Objectives
      1) Gross Revenue
      2) Return on Investment and Desired Profit Margins
      3) Implications of Being in the Fixed Revenue/Variable Expense Business
      4) Pricing Objectives vis-a-vis Competition

   G. Anticipation of Market Trends in the Managed Care Business and Identification of Specific Steps that will be taken to Address these Trends. For example:
      1) Regionalization of Managed Care Business
      2) Blending of Product Lines
      3) Integration of Diverse Delivery System Models
      4) Declining Differentiation Between Indemnity and Managed Care Utilization Patterns
      5) Balancing of Growth, Financial, and Operations Objectives

   H. Development of Effective Means of Resolving Potential Inherent (but not Unresolvable) Conflicts of Interest Between Providers and Managed Care Companies

2. *A clear understanding of the criteria for success in the managed dare business by the board, management, and key hospital and physician leaders*

   A. Specific "Game Plan" Regarding How to Meet the Criteria

   B. Ability to Execute in Timely Fashion

3. *Development of an effective organization structure which:*

   A. Anticipates Growth and Functional Objectives

   B. Maximizes Efficiencies with the Administrative and Marketing, as well as the Provider Support Components of the Organization

   C. Clearly Defines and Delegates Responsibility and Authority for Specific Functions and Objectives

D. Utilizes Standardized and Periodically Updated Operating Policies and Procedures and Corporate Documents (eg, Provider Contracts)

E. Applies Available Technology in Order to Upgrade Service Capabilities (eg, Paperless Claims Systems, Computer Modeled Referral Authorization Systems, etc)

4. *Ability to Recruit and retain competent management and support staff*

A. Competitive Compensation Packages (eg, Base Salaries, Fringe Benefits, and Incentive Plans)

B. Career Enhancement Opportunities

C. Formal training programs

5. *Ability to significantly impact the quality of care, utilization patterns, and unit costs through a properly structured and effectively managed health care delivery system*

A. Selection of Physician Leadership with Specified Qualifications

B. Timely and Objective Quality and Cost Measurement, Management, and Reporting

C. Development of a Provider (Physician, Hospital, etc) Incentive System that is Fair, Relatively Simple, and Effective

D. Proper Recognition of the Role, Value, and Responsibility of the Patient Manager (Primary Care Physician) in the Managed Care Business

E. Careful Provider Screening, Education, and Ongoing Support, which includes:
   1) Accurate and Timely Reporting of Provider Activity that is Properly Summarized, Trended, and Benchmarked
   2) Physician Office Support

F. Particular Focus on Ambulatory Care Management (Assumes Inpatient Component is Already under Control)

G. The Sizing of the HMO Provider Network must Assure a Reasonable Volume of Business for Providers from the Managed Care Company

6. *Access to adequate and reasonably priced capital*

7. *Development and constant updating of marketing and sales strategies supported by qualified marketing management and staff*

Bibliography

A

Abrahams, Ruby. "The social/HMO: case management in an integrated acute and long-term care system. *Caring* 9(8): 30-32, 34, 36-38, 40. August 1990.

Abrams, Rhoda. "Prepayment in community health centers." *Journal of Ambulatory Care Management* 13(4): 33-40. October 1990.

Abramson, Marcy. "Quality: crucial to success of the health care industry." *Quality* 30(2): 14-19. February 1991.

Adams, Dale W. and Collins, Thomas. "Case studies of hospital pharmacist involvement in managed care. Memorial Medical Center." *American Journal of Hospital Pharmacy* 47(10): 2277-80. October 1990.

Adjusted Community Rate: Example of Analysis. Spring House, PA: Health Economics, Inc., 1990.

Adjusted Community Rate: Instructions and Examples From HCFA on TEFRA Risk Contract. Spring House, PA: Health Economics, Inc., 1990.

Akaah, I. P. and Bacherer, R. C. "Integrating a consumer orientation into the planning of HMO programs: an application of conjoint segmentation." *Journal of Health Care Marketing* 3(2): 9-18. Spring 1983.

Aluise, J. J. *The Physician as Manager* (2nd Ed.). New York: Springer-Verlag, 1986.

Aluise, J.; Bradley, D.; and Zelman, B. "Implications for fee-for-service practices affiliated with independent practice associations." *North Carolina Medical Journal.* June 1987.

Aluise, J.; Konrad, T.; and Buckner, B. "Impact of IPAs on fee-for-service medical groups: a case study analysis." *Health Care Management Review.* February 1989.

"Alternative delivery systems." *Health Affairs* 5(1). Spring 1986.

AmbuMed Systems Associates and Technology Management, Inc. *Compendium of Managed Health Care Computer System Vendors.* Silver Spring, MD: Birch & Davis Associates, Inc., 1988.

American Association of Retired Persons. *Choosing an HMO; An Evaluation Checklist.* Washington, DC: AARP, 1986.

Anderson, Donald F. "How effective is managed mental health care? *Business & Health* Special Issue: 13-14. 1990.

Anderson, Gerard F. et al. "Setting payment rates of recapitated systems: a comparison of various alternatives." *Inquiry* 27(3): 225-233. Fall 1990.

Anderson, M. and Dunn, J. "Disclosure of outpatient prescription drug benefits in HMOs." *Health Affairs* 10(2): 143-7. Summer 1991.

Anderson, O. W. et al. *HMO Development: Patterns and Prospects, A Comparative Analysis of HMOs.* Continuing CHAS Research Series - No. 33. Chicago: Pluribus Press, Inc., 1985.

Anonymous. "Administrators move to manage health care." *Employee Benefit Plan Review* 45(7): 28-32. January 1991.

Anonymous. "Managed care industry polices itself through accreditation." *Employee Benefit Plan Review* 46(5). November 1991.

Anonymous. "Managed care plans show signs of maturity." *Employee Benefit Plan Review* 46(5): 30-34. November 1991.

Anonymous. "Planning your health care strategy; wellness, HMOs, and cost control." *Business & Health* Special Issue: 6-8. October 1991.

Ansel, Daniel E. "Behavioral health care: use several criteria to select managed care provider." *Business Insurance* 25(28): 24. July 15, 1991.

Aquilina, David. "The role of MIS in managed care: Managed care challenges of the 1990s." *Medical Interface:* 45, 48-49, 52. April 1990.

Arispe, Irma E. *1991 Sourcebook on HMO Utilization Data.* Washington, DC: GHAA, June 1991.

Arispe, Irma E. *GHAA Survey of Member Plans with Medicaid Contracts: Findings.* Washington, DC: GHAA, July 1990.

Arkans HD. "HMOs today" (editorial). *New Jersey Medicine* 88(6): 395-6. June 1991.

Armour, Eric; Phillips, David; and Lance, Larry K. "Making managed care work: two prescriptions." *National Underwriter (Life/Health/Financial Services)* 95(16): 7, 10, 16, 33. April 22, 1991.

Arnold, W. V. and Leonard, M. "HMOs and PPOs: an operational guide." *Topics in Health Care Financing* 13(3): 19-31. Spring 1987.

B

Bailey, Nancy Coe. "Mental health benefits: breaking through the clouds." *Business & Health* 8(6): 46-58, 60. June 1990.

Banks, Naomi J. and Palmer, R. Heather. "Clinical reminders in ambulatory care." *HMO Practice* 4(4): 131-136. July/August 1990.

Bard, Marc A. "Recruiting physicians: making the right choices." *HMO Practice* 4(6): 220-223. November/December 1990.

Barter, Bruce. "Case management in HMOs." *HMO Practice* 5(1): 1-2. January/February 1991.

Bell, Christy W.; Lewis, Barbara Edelman; and Zelley, Molly O. "Managed care: update and future directions." *Journal of Ambulatory Care Management* 13(2): 15-26. May 1990.

Bell, Clark W. "Success of managed care needs hospital participation." *Modern Healthcare* 20(38): 14. September 24, 1990.

Bergmark, R. and Edward-Parker, Marcie. "Future trends and issues in health care, managed care, and LTC for seniors." *Broker World* 11(5): 46-50, 118. May 1991.

Berkowitz, Edward D. and Wolff, Wendy. *Group Health Association: A Portrait of a Health Maintenance Organization: Health, Society and Policy.* Philadelphia: Temple University Press, 1988.

Berman, Henry and Rose, Louisa. *Choosing the Right Health Care Plan.* Mount Vernon, NY: Consumers Union, 1990.

Berman, Henry S. "The time has come: HMOs and the uninsured." *HMO Practice* 5(2): 55-57. March/April 1991.

Bernstein Research. *Health Maintenance Organizations: Strategic Analysis/Financial Forecast.* New York: Bernstein Research, 1986.

Bernstein Research. *The Future of Health Care Delivery in America.* New York: Sanford C. Bernstein, April 1990.

Bertko, John and Pearman, AnnMarie. "A health plan designed by employees and physicians." *Business & Health* 9(2): 58-61. February 1991.

Berwick, D. M. and Coltin, K. L. "Feedback reduces test use in a health maintenance organization." *Journal of the American Medical Association* 255: 1450-54, 1986.

Berwick D. M. et al. "Performance of a five-item mental health screening test." *Medical Care* 29(2): 169-76. February 1991.

Betty, Warren R. et al. "Physician practice profiles: a valuable information system for HMOs." *Medical Group Management Journal* 37(6): 68-71, 73, 75. November/December 1990.

Bice, Thomas W. "Medicaid and Health Maintenance Organizations: A Review of Selectivity in Enrollment and Disenrollment." *HMOs and Medicaid — New Initiative and Challenges.* Section 3. Denver, Colorado, October 7-8, 1986. Washington, DC: GHAA, 1986.

Bierce A. "HMOs today" (editorial). *New Jersey Medicine* 88(2): 89-90. February 1991.

Birnbaum, R. W. *Health Maintenance Organizations: A Guide to Planning and Development.* Jamaica, NY: Spectrum Publications, 1976.

Black, Jimmy. "Management and compliance strategy for a prescription drug formulary in an IPA-model HMO." *Drug Benefit Trends* 2(4): 7-10. July-August 1990.

Bledsoe, Turner. "Physician assistants and nurse practitioners: needed more than ever." *HMO Practice* 4(5): 155-156. September/October 1990.

Block, Lori. "Employers differ on the success of managed care." *Business Insurance* 25(38): 21-25. September 23, 1991.

Bloom, Alan. "Liability concerns in the design of HMO UR/QA Programs." *Risk Management in Managed Health Care Systems.* Section 3. Washington, DC, December 3-5, 1986. Washington, DC: GHAA, 1986.

Bloom, Jill. *HMOs: What They Are, How They Work, and Which One Is Best for You.* Tucson, AZ: Body Press, 1987.

Bodewes, Cynthia A. et al. "Meeting the challenge of managed care." *Medical Group Management Journal* 38(1): 44-46. January-February 1991.

Boland, Peter (ed.) *Making Managed Healthcare Work: A Practical Guide to Strategies and Solutions.* Rockville, MD: Aspen Publications, 1991.

Boland, Peter (ed.) *The New Healthcare Market: A Guide to PPOs for Purchasers, Payors, and Providers.* Homewood, Illinois: Dow Jones-Irwin, 1985.

Bozman, Jean S. "VAX system helps HMO improve patient care." *Computerworld* 25(14): 29. April 8, 1991.

Bradbury, Robert C.; Golec, Joseph H.; and Stearns, Frank E. "Comparing hospital length of stay in independent practice association HMOs and traditional insurance programs." *Inquiry* 28(1): 87-93. Spring 1991.

Bradford, Larry. "Quality of service: a new paradigm for managed health care." *Medical Interface* 3(12): 27-28, 31, 37. December 1990.

Bradley, Susan; Shadle-Peterson, Maureen; and Hunter, Mary M. *1990 National Managed Care Firms.* Excelsior, MN: InterStudy, March 1991.

Brant, Owen. "From mini to mainframe: How one HMO made the leap." *Computers in Healthcare:* 26-28. September 1990.

Breivis, James S. "The specialist in the HMO." *HMO Practice* 4(6): 211-214. November/December 1990.

A Brief Look at Managed Care. Silver Spring, MD: National Association of Social Workers, October 1990.

Brock, C. B. "Consultation and referral patterns of family physicians." *The Journal of Family Practice* 4(4): 1129-1134. 1977.

Brody, H. "Cost containment as professional challenge." *Theoretical Medicine* 8: 5-17. 1987

Brostoff, Steven. "State mandates on managed care hike costs: study." *National Underwriter (Life/Health/Financial Services)* 95(33): 2. August 19, 1991.

Bucci, Michael. "Health maintenance organizations: plan offerings and enrollments." *Monthly Labor Review* 114(4): 11-18. April 1991.

Buckner, J. "The managed care marketplace." *Journal of Health Care Marketing* 10(1): 2-5. March 1990.

Burakoff, Ronald P. "Dentistry and health maintenance organizations." *Special Care in Dentistry* 8(4): 163-6. July-August 1990.

Burda, David. "Hospitals' managed-care alliances investigated." *Modern Healthcare* 21(15): 20. April 15, 1991.

Burke, Terrence C. "Making managed care work for you." *Health Systems Review* 24(3): 12-14. May/June 1991.

Burke, Thomas P. and Jain, Rita S. "Trends in employer-provided health care benefits." *Monthly Labor Review* 114(2): 24-30. February 1991.

C

Cabin, William D. *A Primer on Managed Care of the Home Care Industry.* Mishawaka, IN: William D. Cabin, Health Care Consultant, 1985.

Calise, Angela K. "PPOs called a cure for workers' comp. woes." *National Underwriter (Property/Casualty/Employee Benefits)* 95(28): 10. July 15, 1991.

Cappabiance, Edward C. "Mental health benefits in HMOs." *Drug Benefit Trends* 2(4): 10-14. July/August 1990.

Carey, Tim; Weis, Kathi; and Homer, Charles. "Prepaid versus traditional medicaid plans: effects on preventive health care." *Journal of Clinical Epidemiology* 43(11): 1213-1220. November 1990.

"Caring for the uninsured and underinsured. Special issue." *Journal of the American Medical Association* 265(19): 2441-2576. May 15, 1991.

Carroll, Lisa. "Providing health coverage for America's small business community: Opportunities for HMOs." *Medical Interface* 3(12): 32-33, 36-37. December 1990.

Cascardo, Debra. "Factors affecting cost containment in an HMO: a review of the literature." *Journal of Ambulatory Care Management* 5(3): 53-63. August 1982.

Cassel C. "Doctors and allocation decisions: a new role in the new medicine." *Journal of Health Politics, Policy, and Law,* 10: 549-64. 1985.

Cautions for Prepaid Organized Health Care Under a National Health System: Lessons From Canada. Washington, DC: GHAA, February 1990.

"Cautious partners: interview with HCFA administrator Gail Wilensky." *HMO Magazine* 31(6): 9-11. November/December 1990.

Cavaiani, Ralph P. and Bartlein, Barbara A. "Implementing a combined EAP/managed care program for mental health and substance abuse services." *Medical Interface* 4(1): 19-20, 22-23. January 1991.

Chandler, Ralph P. and Carr, Susan L. "Making a difference: the pharmaceutical-managed care partnership." *Medical Interface* 3(5): 22-24, 26. May 1990.

Chenen, Arthur R. "Harrell v. total health care: the corporate responsibility doctrine applies to managed care providers." *The Medical Staff Counselor* 4(3): 61-63. Summer 1990.

Childs, Bill W. "Kaiser Permanente's success story." *Healthcare Informatics* 7(8): 26-28. August 1990.

Christensen, Lynne. "The highs and lows of PPOs." *Business & Health* 9(9): 72-77. September 1991.

Christianson, Jon B. et al. "The HMO industry: evolution in population demographics and market structures." *Medical Care Review* 48(1): 3-46. Spring 1991.

Coddington, Dean C.; Keen, David J.; and Moore, Keith D. "Cost shifting overshadows employers' cost-containment efforts." *Business & Health* 9(1): 45-46, 48, 50-51. January 1991.

Coile, R. C. Jr. "Managed care: 10 leading trends for the 1990s: Part I." *Aspen's Advisor for the Nurse Executive* 5(6): 4-5, 7. March 1990.

Coile, Russell C. Jr. *The New Medicine: Reshaping Medical Practice and Healthcare Delivery.* Rockville, MD: Aspen Publishers, 1990.

Coleman, J. R. and Kaminsky, F. C. *Designing Medical Services for Health Maintenance Organizations.* (Volume IV in a Series: Ambulatory Care Systems.) Lexington, MA: Lexington Books, 1977.

Comparing Health Systems: An Internal Survey of Consumer Satisfaction. Boston, MA: Harvard Community Health Plan & Louis Harris and Associates, 1991.

Comparing Health Systems: An International Survey of Consumer Satisfaction. Boston, MA: Harvard Community Health Plan & Louis Harris and Associates, 1991.

Considine J. M. and Oakes L. S. "HMOs: survival of the fittest." *New Jersey Medicine* 88(2): 111-4. February 1991

Contracting Guidelines for Internists. American Society of Internal Medicine, 1101 Vermont Avenue, NW, Suite 500, Washington, DC 20005-3547.

Cook, J. and Rodnick, J. "Evaluating HMO/IPA contracts for family physicians: one group's experience." *Journal of Family Practice* 26(3): 325-331. 1988.

Corcoran, Maureen E. "Employers may face increased liability for managed care." *Journal of Compensation & Benefits* 6(6): 47-48. May/June 1991.

Corrigan, Janet M. and Thompson, Laurie M. "Involvement of health maintenance organizations in graduate medical education." *Academic Medicine* 66(11): 656-661. November 1991.

Cotterell C. C.; Dombroske L.; and Fischermann E. A. "Comprehensive drug-use evaluation program in a health maintenance organization." *American Journal of Hospital Pharmacy* 48(8): 1712-7. August 1991.

Council on Medical Service. "Guidelines for Quality Assurance." *Journal of the American Medical Association* 259: 2572-73.

Cox, Brian. "Enrollment in open-ended HMOs soared in 1990." *National Underwriter (Life/Health/Financial Services)* 95(42): 2, 8. October 21, 1991.

Cox, Brian. "Know competition in marketing HMOS, PPOs." *National Underwriter (Property/Casualty/Employee Benefits)* 95(30): 11, 39. July 29, 1991.

Cox, Brian. "Sears installing managed care plan." *National Underwriter (Property/Casualty/Employee Benefits)* 95(20): 13, 15. May 20, 1991.

Coyne, Joseph S. and Meadows, David M. "California HMOs may provide national forecast." *Healthcare Financial Management* 45(5): 34-39. May 1991.

Craig, Paul. "Health maintenance organization gatekeeping policies: Potential liability for deterring access to emergency medical services." *Journal of Health and Hospital Law* 23(5): 135-46. May 1990.

Creed, Barbara B.; Corcoran, Maureen E.; and Leitner, Marcia. "Managing the legal risks of managed care programs." *Pension World* 27(8): 14-16. August 1991.

Crosson, Cynthia. "Managed care cos. more exposed to legal liability." *National Underwriter (Life/Health/Financial Services)* 95(18): 3, 5. May 6, 1991.

Crosson, Cynthia. "Managed care sales create new world at CIGNA." *National Underwriter (Life/Health/Financial Services)* 95(22): 14, 20. June 3, 1991.

Crosson, Cynthia. "Pru unveils PPO in 43 locations nationwide." *National Underwriter (Life/Health/Financial Services)* 95(4): 11. January 28, 1991.

Crump W. J. and Massengill, P. "Outpatient consultations from a family practice residency program: nine years' experience." *Journal of the American Board of Family Practice,* 1(3).

Cunningham, F. C. and Williamson, J. W. "How does the quality of health care in HMOs compare to that in other settings? An analytic literature review: 1958-1979." *Group Health Journal* 1(1): 4-25. Winter 1980.

Currey, Wesley. "Status quo won't work. (Interview of Joe Duva.)" *Physician Executive* 16(4): 2-5. July-August 1990.

Curtiss, Frederic R. "Managed care: the second generation." *American Journal of Hospital Pharmacy* 47(9): 2047-2052. September 1990.

D

Dalton, John J. "Alternative delivery systems and employers." *Topics in Health Care Financing* 13(3): 68-76. Spring 1987.

Davies, A. R. et al. "Consumer acceptance of prepaid and fee-for-service medical care: results from a randomized controlled trial (Rand Study)." *Health Services Research* 21(3): 431-452. August 1986.

Davis, Aubrey. "The role of Group Health Cooperative in the development of Washington State's basic health plan." *Henry Ford Hospital Medical Journal* 38(2-3): 128-9. 1990.

Davis, Gary Scott. "Introduction: managed health care primer." In: *The Insider's Guide to Managed Care: A Legal and Operational Roadmap*, pp. 13-35. Washington, DC: NHLA, 1990.

Defino, Theresa. "Small business looms large." *HMO Magazine* 32(2): 24-28. March/April 1991.

DeFuria, Maureen C. and Shimshak, Daniel G. "Analyzing and measuring disenrollment/enrollment: practical application of the theory." *Medical Interface* 3(10): 44, 46-48. October 1990.

DeFuria, Maureen C. and Shimshak, Daniel G. "Analyzing and measuring disenrollment/enrollment: the theory behind health plan choice models." *Medical Interface* 3(9): 14, 16, 21, 22, 25. September 1990.

Del Toro, Iris M. "Designing chemical dependency programs in HMOs." *HMO Practice* 4(1): 19-23. January/February 1990.

Dellinger, Anne M. (ed.) *Healthcare facilities law : critical issues for hospitals, HMOs, and extended care facilities.* Boston: Little, Brown, 1991.

DeMarco, W. J. and Garvey, T. J. *Going prepaid: a strategic planning decision.* (A monograph in the Going Prepaid Series). Denver, CO: Center for Research in Ambulatory Health Care Administration, Medical Group Management Association, 1986.

DeMarco, William J. and Traska, Maria R. *Physician Payment Reform: Why Its Time Has Come.* 3v Rockford, IL: Warren Surveys, 1991.

Dietrich, A. J. et al. "Do primary physicians actually manage their patients' fee-for-service care?" *Journal of the American Medical Association* 259: 3145-3149. 1988.

Diosegy, Arlene J. "Managed care contracts. Dangerous liaisons?" *North Carolina Medical Journal* 51(10): 534-6. October 1990.

Dolinsky, A. L. and Caputo R. K. "An assessment of employers' experiences with HMOs: factors that make a difference." *Health Care Management Review* 16(1): 25-31. Winter 1991.

Dolinsky, Arthur L. and Caputo, Richard K. "An assessment of employers' experiences with HMOs: factors that make a difference." *Health Marketing Quarterly* 8(1-2): 31-43. 1990.

Dolinsky, Arthur L. and Caputo, Richard K. "Intentions to join HMOs: perceived relative performance versus satisfaction/dissatisfaction." *Journal of Hospital Marketing* 4(2): 135-48. 1990.

Dolinsky, Arthur L. and Caputo, Richard K. "The role of health care attributes and demographic characteristics in the determination of health care satisfaction." *Journal of Health Care Marketing* 10(4): 31-9. December 1990.

Donabedian A. "The quality of care: how can it be assessed?" *Journal of the American Medical Association* 260: 2743-48. 1988.

"Does IPA-provider contract exclude provider's competitors?" *HealthSpan* 7(1): 22. January 1990.

Dragalin, D.; Perkins, D.; and Plocher, D. W. "Institutes of quality: Prudential's approach to outcomes management for specialty procedures." *Quality Review Bulletin* 16(3): 111-5. March 1990.

Drew, Judith C. "Health maintenance organizations: history, evolution and survival." *Nursing and Health Care* 11(3): 144-149. March 1990.

Ducharme, Barbara K.; Lowenhaupt, Manuel T.; and Holland, Chris T. "Getting a fix on the office." *HMO Magazine* 32(3): 53-54, 60. May/June 1991.

Dunmire, Susen N. "Health care delivery systems in review." *Journal of Medical Practice Management* 5(3): 195-196. Winter 1990.

Dunston, Janice. "How managed care can work for you." *Nursing* 20(10): 56-9. October 1990.

Durfee, Donna and Patchett, Jeffery A. "Case studies of hospital pharmacist involvement in managed care. Presbyterian Hospital." *American Journal of Hospital Pharmacy* 47(10): 2280-3. October 1990.

Durkee, Ray. "Total quality management in managed care: a special challenge of the 1990s." *Medical Interface* 4(3): 11-12, 21. March 1991.

Duva, Joseph W. "Shared-risk arrangement between employers and insurers." *American Journal of Hospital Pharmacy* 47(9): 2056-2059. September 1990.

E

Ebert, R. H. "Has the acute general hospital become an inappropriate environment for the education of the primary care physician?" *Journal of Laboratory & Clinical Medicine* 117(6): 438-42. June 1991.

Eidus, Robert and Warburton, Samuel W. (eds.) *Managed Health Care: A Teaching Syllabus.* Kansas City, MO: Society of Teachers of Family Medicine, May 1990.

Elgin, Peggie R. "Managed Care Plan Cuts $20 Million from Utility's Health Bills." *Corporate Cashflow* 12(1): 18, 20. January 1991.

Elliott, Thomas E.; Dunaye, Thomas M.; and Johnson, Paulette M. "Determining patient satisfaction in a Medicare health maintenance organization." *Journal of Ambulatory Care Management* 4(1): 34-46. January 1991.

Ellsbury, Kathleen. "A Primary Physician's Guide to HMOs." STFM reprint service.

Ellwein, L. K.; Malcolm, J.; and Shandle, M. *Hospital Sponsored HMOs.* Excelsior, MN: Interstudy, 1982.

Enthoven, A. C. "The Rand experiment and economical health care." *New England Journal of Medicine* 310(23): 1528-1530. June 7, 1984.

Enthoven, Alain C. *Theory and Practice of Managed Competition in Health Care Finance.* Amsterdam; New York: Science Pub. Co., 1988.

Epstein, Steven B.; Lutes, Mark, Shapiro-Snyder, Lynn. "The new threat to managed care." *Best's Review (Life/Health)* 92(6): 67-70, 138-139. October 1991.

Ermann, Dan. "Health maintenance organizations: the future of the for-profit plan." *Journal of Ambulatory Care Management* 9(2): 72-84. May 1986.

Executive Compensation Institute. *1990/91 Managed Care Executive Pay/Board Practices Study: 6th Edition.* Moss Beach, CA: Executive Compensation Institute/J. Richard & Co., 1991.

Executive Compensation Institute. *1991 Managed Care Study of Executive Compensation and Staffing Ratios.* Moss Beach, CA: Executive Compensation Institute/J. Richard & Co., May 1991.

Executive Managed Care Directory. A Comprehensive Reference to Managed Care Suppliers and Plans. 1991-1992 edition. Bronxville, NY: Medical Interface, 1991.

"Expert: managed care plans should be sensitive to industry trends to understand legal climate." *Managed Care Law Outlook Special Report* 2(7): 1-8. July 1990.

F

Falk C. D. "Our HMO offers more than medical care." *Rn* 54(9): 17-8. September 1991.

Faltermayer, Edmund. "Strong medicine for health costs." *Fortune* 121(9): 221, 224, 226, 227, 230. April 23, 1990.

Family Practice and the Managed Care Industry: Issues and Answers. Proceedings of an AAFP Conference, June 2-3, 1987.

Fant, David J. and Pool, Christopher J. "The CHAMPUS reform initiative and fiscal intermediary managed care." *Journal of Ambulatory Care Management* 13(3): 22-28. July 1990.

Feldman, Roger et al. "Effects of HMOs on the creation of competitive markets for hospital services." *Journal of Health Economics* 9(2): 207-222. September 1990.

Feldstein, Adrianne; Vollmer, William; and Valanis, Barbara. "Evaluating the patient-handling tasks of nurses." *Journal of Occupational Medicine* 32(10). October 1990.

Fine, Allan. "Consultative selling: taking careful aim at managed care." *Medical Interface* 3(7): 37-38, 52. July 1990.

Fine, J. S. "The practice of adolescent medicine in staff model HMOs." *HMO Practice* 3(1): 16-21. January-February 1989.

Fink P. J. and Dubin W. R. "No free lunch: limitations on psychiatric care in HMOs." *Hospital & Community Psychiatry* 42(4): 363-5. April 1991.

Finkler M. D. and Wirtschafter D. D. "Cost-effectiveness and obstetric services." *Medical Care* 29(10): 951-63. October 1991.

Fischer, Lucy Rose et al. "How does an HMO decide whether to create its own home health care agency or contract out for services?" *Health Care Supervisor* 9(3): 39-50. April 1991.

Ford, John L. "Enrollment forecasting in the largest HMOs: an exploratory descriptive study." *Medical Interface* 4(1): 14-16, 23. January 1991.

Forstrom, M. J. et al. "Effect of a clinical pharmacist program on the cost of hypertension treatment in an HMO family practice clinic." *Drug Intelligence and Clinical Pharmacy* 24(3): 304-309. March 1990.

Fox, Harriette B. et al. *An Examination of HMO Policies Affecting Children With Special Needs.* Washington, DC: Fox Health Policy Consultants, Inc. September 1990.

Fox, Peter D. "Tailor-made elder care." *HMO Magazine* 32(1): 25-29. January/February 1991.

Fox, Peter D. and Anderson, M. D. "Hybrid HMOs, PPOs: the new focus." *Business and Health* 3(4): 20, 21, 24, 26, 26. March 1986.

Fox, Peter D. and Steele, Richard J. *Determinants of HMO Success.* Rockville, MD: US DHHS, OHMO, January 1986.

Fox, Peter D. et al. *Initiatives in Service Delivery for the Elderly in HMOs.* Washington, DC: Lewin/ICF, February 1991.

Freeborn, Donald K. et al. "Consistently high users of medical care among the elderly." *Medical Care* 28(6): 527-540. June 1990.

Frieden, Joyce. "PPO review: will it tell employers what they want to know?" *Business & Health* 8(6): 30, 34, 36, 38. June 1990.

Frieden, Joyce. "The 1991 premium forecast." *Business & Health* 9(1): 55. January 1991.

Fritz, Dan and Repko, David V. "A blueprint for forging new HMO relationships." *Business and Health.* 3(8): 38, 39. July/August 1986.

Froom, J.; Feinbloom, R. I.; and Rosen, M. G. "Risk of Referral." *Journal of Family Practice* 18(4): 623-626. 1987.

G

Gajda, Anthony J. "New cost control opportunities with managed health care." *Journal of Compensation & Benefits* 6(4): 12-18. January/February 1991.

Garcia-Bryce, Ariadna. "Plan would extend capitation to non-HMOs." *Internist* 31(7): 31. July/August 1990.

Garlitz, Glaudia J. "A managed care check-up." *HMO Magazine* 32(2): 6-7. March/April 1991.

Geisel, Jerry. "Employers cite PPO effectiveness." *Business Insurance* 25(32): 1, 78-79. August 12, 1991.

Geisel, Jerry. "HMO savings confirmed - PPOs also reduce costs, survey finds." *Business Insurance* 25(32): 79. August 12, 1991.

Geisel, Jerry. "If managed care fails, is it 'O Canada' for US?" *Business Insurance* 25(38): 28. September 23, 1991.

Geisel, Jerry. "Open-ended HMOs catch on." *Business Insurance* 25(37): 1, 97. September 16, 1991.

GHAA Legislative Dept. and GHAA Legal Dept. *Legislative & Regulatory Issues Digest.* Washington, DC: GHAA, Spring 1991.

GHAA Research and Analysis Department. *HMO Industry Profile: Volume 1: Benefits, Premiums, and Market Structure in 1988.* Washington, DC: GHAA, June 1989.

GHAA Research and Analysis Department. *HMO Industry Profile: Volume 2: Utilization Patterns, 1987*. Washington, DC: GHAA, September 1989.

GHAA Research and Analysis Department. *HMO Industry Profile: Volume 3: Financial Performance, 1987*. Washington, DC: GHAA, December 1989.

GHAA Research and Analysis Dept. *Patterns in HMO Enrollment*. Washington, DC: GHAA, June 1991.

GHAA state legislative and regulatory survey for 1990. Washington, DC: GHAA, 1991.

GHAA. *Clinical Staffing in Prepaid Group Practice HMOs*. Proceedings of the Medical Directors Conference, 5(2). Minneapolis, MN. October 24-25, 1980. Washington, DC GHAA, 1980.

GHAA. *Financial Management Tools for Group Practice HMO Medical Directors and Physician Managers*. Proceedings of the Medical Directors Conference, 6(3). Washington, DC January 8-9, 1982. Washington, DC GHAA, 1982.

GHAA. *GHAA's 1987 Survey of HMO Industry Trends*. Washington, DC GHAA, 1987.

GHAA. *GHAA's Legislative and Regulatory Issues Digest*. Washington, DC GHAA, 1987.

GHAA. *GHAA's National Directory of HMOs*. Washington, DC GHAA, 1987.

GHAA. *HMOs Confronting New Challenges: 1985 Group Health Proceedings*. San Diego, California June 2-5, 1985. Washington, DC GHAA, 1985.

GHAA. *HMOs in a New Era of Health Benefits: 1984 Group Health Proceedings*. Philadelphia, PA. June 10-13, 1984. Washington, DC GHAA, 1984.

GHAA. *HMOs Physicians Managing HMO Physicians*. Proceedings of the Medical Directors Conference 5(6). Denver, CO. February 13-14, 1981. Washington, DC GHAA, 1981.

GHAA. *Hospital Contracting in Group Practice HMOs*. Proceedings of the Medical Directors Conference, 6(1). Washington, DC June 12-13, 1981. Washington, DC: GHAA, 1981.

GHAA. *New Health Care Systems: HMOs and Beyond: 1986 Group Health Proceedings*. Minneapolis, MN. June 1-4, 1986. Washington, DC GHAA, 1986.

GHAA. *Utilization Management Techniques in Prepaid Group Practice Health Maintenance Organization*. Washington, DC GHAA, 1983.

Gifford, Gregory et al. "A simultaneous equations model of employer strategies for controlling health benefit costs." *Inquiry* 28(1): 56-66. Spring 1991.

Gilman, Thomas A. and Bucco, Cynthia K. "Alternative Delivery Systems: An Overview." *Topics in Health Care Financing* 13(3): 1-7. Spring 1987.

Ginsburg, Paul B. et al. *Research Plan for the Preferred Provider Organization Study*. Prepared for the US Department of Health and Human Services. Santa Monica, CA: Rand Corp, 1986.

Ginsburg, William H. "Liability in limbo." *HMO Magazine* 31(4): 23-24. July/August 1990.

Glaser, Martha. "Managed care bites benefit!" *Business & Health* 9(5): 71-72, 74, 76, 78. May 1991.

Glenn, J. K.; Lawler, F. H.; and Hoerl, M. S. "Physician referrals in a competitive environment: an estimate of the economic impact of a referral." *Journal of the American Medical Association* 258: 1920-1923. 1987.

"Glossary." *HealthWeek* 4(4): 37. February 26, 1990.

Glossary of Managed Health Care Terms. Minnetonka, MN: United HealthCare Corporation, December 1990.

Gold, M. "Health maintenance organizations: structure, performance, and current issues for employee health benefits design." *Journal of Occupational Medicine* 33(3): 288-96. March 1991.

Gold, Marsha and Camerlo, Kevin. *1991 Premium Rates and Employee Costs Within the Federal Employees Health Benefits Program, and Trends, 1988-1991*. Washington, DC: GHAA, November 1990.

Gold, Marsha and Camerlo, Kevin. *HMO Market Position Report: Results From an October 1990 Member Plan Survey*. Washington, DC: GHAA, November 1990.

Gold, Marsha and Camerlo, Kevin. *HMO Market Position Report: Results From a Fall 1991 Member Plan Survey*. Washington, DC: GHAA, December 1991.

Gold, Marsha and Camerlo, Kevin. *Update on the 1990 Premium Rates and Employee Costs Within the Federal Employees Health Benefits Program*. Washington, DC: GHAA, December 1989.

Gold, Marsha and Hodges, Dennis. GHAA Research and Analysis Department. *HMO Industry Profile: Vol. 1: Benefits, Premiums, and Market Structure in 1990*. Washington, DC: GHAA, June 1991.

Gold, Marsha and Hodges, Dennis. *HMO Industry Profile: Volume 1: Benefits, Premiums and Market Structure in 1989*. Washington, DC: GHAA, June 1990.

Gold, Marsha and Hodges, Dennis. *HMO Industry Profile; Volume 1: Benefits, Premiums, and Market Structure in 1990*. Washington, DC: GHAA, June 1990.

Gold, Marsha R. "HMOs and managed care." *Health Affairs* 10(4): 189-206. Winter 1991.

Gold, Marsha; Hodges, Dennis; and Camerlo, Kevin. *HMO Market Position Report: Results of a November 1989 Member Plan Survey*. Washington, DC: GHAA, December 1989.

Goldberg, Lawrence S. "HMOs and CMPs: federal regulations." *Topics in Health Care Financing* 13(3): 38-46. Spring 1987.

Goldfield, Norbert and Goldsmith, Seth B. (eds.) *Alternative Delivery Systems*. Rockville, MD: Aspen Publications, 1986.

Goldman, Harold B. "When patients complain." *HMO Practice* 5(2): 51-54. March/April 1991.

Goldman, L.; Lee, T.; and Rudd, P. "Ten commandments for effective consultations." *Archives of Internal Medicine* 143: 1753-1755. September 1982.

Gravdal, J. A.; Krohm C.; and Glasser M. "Payment mechanism and patterns of use of medical services: the example of hypertension." *Journal of Family Practice* 32(1): 66-70. January 1991.

Gray, Wendy B. *Implementing Managed Health Care*. New York: Conference Board, 1991.

Grazier, Kyle L. et al. "Factors affecting choice of health care plans." Health Services Research 20(6): 659-682. February 1986.

Greenberg, Warren. *Response to AIDS in the Private Sector: Case Studies of HMOs, Insurers and Employers*. Alexandria, VA: Capital Publishing Group, January 1989.

Greenlich, Merwyn R.; Freeborn, Donald K.; and Pope, Clyde R. (eds.) *Health care research in an HMO: Two decades of discovery*. Baltimore: Johns Hopkins University Press, 1988.

Greenlick, Merwyn R.; Freeborn, Donald K.; and Pope, Clyde R. (eds.) *Health Care Research in an HMO: Two Decades of Discovery*. The Johns Hopkins Series in Contemporary Medicine & Public Health. Baltimore, MD: Johns Hopkins University Press, 1988.

Greer, James A. Jr. "Distribution of prepaid income." *Physician Executive* 16(6): 30-32. November/December 1990.

Griffin, Teresa. "Texas HMOs and PPOs: coming on strong in the '90s." *Texas Medical Journal* 86(9): 67-9. September 1990.

Grizzard, M. B.; Harris G.; and Karns H. "Use of outpatient parenteral antibiotic therapy in a health maintenance organization." *Reviews of Infectious Diseases* 13 Suppl 2: S174-9. January-February 1991.

Grossman, Woodrin. "Risk contracting." *Topics in Health Care Financing* 16(4): 24-31. Summer 1990.

Gruber, Lynn et al. *The Bottom Line: HMO Premiums and Profitability, 1988-1989*. Excelsior, MN: InterStudy, 1989.

Gruber, Lynn et al. *The Interstudy Edge 1990, Volume 2*. Excelsior, MN: InterStudy, 1990.

Gruber, Lynn et al. *The InterStudy Edge. Volume 1*. Excelsior, MN: InterStudy, 1990.

Gruber, Lynn et al. *The InterStudy Edge. Volume 2*. Excelsior, MN: InterStudy, 1989.

Gruber, Lynn; Shadle, Maureen; and Pion, Kirk. *The InterStudy Edge 1989. Volume 4*. Excelsior, MN: Interstudy, 1989.

Guay, A. H. "Managed dental care—coming soon to your neighborhood." *Journal of the Connecticut State Dental Association* 67(1): 17-22. Spring 1991.

Guide for Fee-for-Service Medical Groups on Affiliation with HMOs. Rockville, MD: Dept. of Health and Human Services, Public Health Service, Health Resources and Services Administration, 1983.

H

Hahn, Susan M. and Kleinke, J. D. "Managed mental health for the 1990s: integrating managed care and employee assistance." *Compensation & Benefits Management* 7(4): 1-6. Fall 1991.

Halvorson, George C. "There are additional lessons to be learned." *Group Practice Journal* 39(4): 19, 26, 30. July/August 1990.

Hansell, S.; Sherman G.; and Mechanic D. "Body awareness and medical care utilization among older adults in an HMO." *Journal of Gerontology* 46(3): S151-9. May 1991.

Hansen, J. P. et al. "Factors related to an effective referral and consultation process." *Journal of Family Practice* 15(4): 651-656. 1982.

A harder look at health care costs. Conference presentations edited by Melissa A. Berman. New York: Conference Board, 1988.

Harrington, Charlene and Newcomer, Robert J. "Social health maintenance organizations' service use and costs, 1985-89." *Health Care Financing Review* 12(3): 37-52. Spring 1991.

Harris, John M. Jr. *The Role of the Medical Director in the Fee-For-Service/Prepaid Medical Group*. (A monograph in the *Going Prepaid* Series). Denver, CO: Center for Research in Ambulatory Health Care Administration, Medical Group Management Association, 1983.

Harty, Sara J. "Companies employ managed care in mental health plans." *Business Insurance* 25(34): 3, 22. August 26, 1991.

Health Care Financing Administration. *The Relationship Between Marketing Strategies and Risk Selection in Medicare At-Risk HMOs*. Ann Arbor, MI: University of Michigan, March 1990.

Health Committee of the Actuarial Standards Board. *Actuarial Practice Concerning Health Maintenance Organizations and Other Managed-Care Health Plans*. Washington, DC: Actuarial Standards Board, July 1990.

Health Managers Letter. Washington, DC: GHAA, 1990.

Heartland Health Plan: An Illustrative Case Study in Approaches to Adjusted Community Rates. Spring House, PA: Health Economics, Inc., 1990.

Heinen, LuAnn; Fox, Peter D.; and Anderson Maren D. "Findings from the Medicaid competition demonstrations: a guide for states." *Health Care Financing Review* 11(4): 55-67. Summer 1990.

Henderson, John A. "Health maintenance organization industry characteristic, trends and market projections." *Health Industry Today* 42-48. August 1985.

Henkoff, Ronald. "Yes, companies can cut health costs." *Fortune* 124(1): 52-56. July 1, 1991.

Herrle, Gregory N. and Alexander, Ralph D. *Considerations in the Design of Open-Ended HMO Products*. Milwaukee, WI: Milliman & Robertson, July 1989.

Herrle, Gregory N. and Pollock, William M. "Multispecialty groups: will they survive prepaid managed care?" *Medical Group Management Journal* 38(1): 24-30. January/February 1991.

Herrle, Gregory N.; Pollock, William M.; and Roberts, Stanley A. *HMO Experience Rating*. Brookfield, WI: Milliman & Robertson, July 1989.

Herrmann, J. "Insurer view: James P. Murphy." *Federation of American Health Systems Review* 23(6): 36. November/December 1990.

Herrmann, John. "Voluntary guidelines for managed care." *Federation of American Health Systems* 23(1): 37-40. January/February 1990.

Hillman, Alan L. "Disclosing information and treating patients as customers." *HMO Practice* 5(2): 37-41. March/April 1991.

Hilsenrath, Peter E. "Managed care and the reorganization of Navy medicine." *Military Medicine* 155(12). December 1990.

Hiramatsu, Sandra. "Member satisfaction in a staff-model health maintenance organization." *American Journal of Hospital Pharmacy* 47(10): 2270-3. October 1990.

"HMO acquisitions seen recovering in 1991, with local deals favored." *Health Market Survey* 8(2): 1, 3-7. January 29, 1991.

"HMO in N.H. to manage HMO in Syracuse, N.Y." *Modern Healthcare* 20(22): 37. June 4, 1990.

"HMO industry structure not likely to change dramatically in 1990s." *Health Market Survey* 7(1): 6-9. January 9, 1990.

HMO Investor's Handbook & Securities Pricing Guide. New York: The Wadsworth Company, 1991.

"HMO penetration passes 15% of US population, keeps rising." *Health Market Survey* 8(3): 3-4. February 18, 1991.

"HMO salary trends." *HMO Magazine* 32(2): 35-36. March/April 1991.

"HMOs' and PPOs' role in health benefits." *Business & Health* 8(6): 8-9. June 1990.

Hodges, Dennis; Camerlo, Kevin; and Gold, Marsha. *HMO Industry Profile: Volume 2: Physician Staffing and Utilization*. Washington, DC: GHAA, August 1990.

Hodges, Dennis; Camerlo, Kevin; and Gold, Marsha. *HMO Industry Profile: Volume 2: Utilization Patterns, 1988*. Washington, DC: GHAA, September 1990.

Holmes, Dari et al. *Nation's HMO Firms 1985*. Excelsior, MN: Interstudy, 1986.

Holoweiko, Mark. "When an HMO takes the rap for a non-member doctor." *Medical Economics* 67(14): 150, 152-154, passim. July 23, 1990.

Hooker, Roderick S. and Freeborn, Donald K. "Use of physician assistants in a managed health care system." *Public Health Reports* 106(1): 90-94. January/February 1991.

Horn, David M. "Successful managed care — a team effort." *Broker World* 11(10): 96-102, 160-161. October 1991.

Horwitz, Sarah McCue and Stein, Ruth E. "Health maintenance organizations vs indemnity insurance of children with chronic illness. Trading gaps in coverage." *American Journal of Disease in Children* 144(5): 581-586. May 1990.

"How do physician assistants practice in you HMO?" *HMO Practice* 4(5): 167-168. September/October 1990.

"How does your plan provide case management?" *HMO Practice* 5(1): 11-13. January/February 1991.

"How has your HMO responded to AIDS?" *HMO Practice* 4(4): 122-123. July/August 1990.

Hreachmack, C. Patrick. "Managed care and EAPs: the right service at the right time!" *Professional Counselor* 5(5): 48. March/April 1991.

Hughes, Edward F. X. (ed.) *Perspectives on Quality in American Health Care*. Washington, DC: McGraw-Hill, 1988.

Hughes, Thomas F. and Eckel, Fred M. "Ethical issues associated with managed care pharmacy services." *Topics in Hospital Pharmacy Management* 10(3): 30-8. November 1990.

Hunter, Mary M. and Shadle, Maureen. *HMOs and Medicare*. Excelsior, MN: Interstudy, 1983.

Hurley, Robert E.; Freund, Deborah A.; and Gage, Barbara J. "Gatekeeper effects on patterns of physician use." *Journal of Family Practice* 32(2): 167-174. February 1991.

I

Iglehart, John K. "Medicare turns to HMOs." *New England Journal of Medicine* 312(20): 132-136. January 10, 1985.

The Insider's Guide to Managed Care: A Legal and Operational Roadmap. NHLA Education in Print Series. Washington, DC: National Health Lawyers Association (NHLA), 1990.

"Interview: strength from within. (Interview with James Walworth.)" *HMO Magazine* 31(3): 9-11. May-June 1990.

The IPA Alternative. American Society of Internal Medicine, 1101 Vermont Avenue, NW, Suite 500, Washington, DC 20005-3547.

InterStudy Quality Edge. Excelsior, MN: InterStudy, 1991.

Interstudy. *1986 June Update: A Midyear Report on HMO Growth*. Excelsior, MN: Interstudy, 1986.

Interstudy. *Hospital Utilization in HMOs*. Excelsior, MN: Interstudy, 1984.

Investors Guide to Health Maintenance Organizations. Washington, DC Government Printing Office, 1982. (GPO Stock #017-002-00153-4).

Isaacs, Florence. *Health Insurance Today: a Consumer Guide to Coverage in the '90s*. Chicago: Blue Cross Shield Association, 1990.

Iverson, Laura H. and Polich, Cynthia, L. *1986 Midyear Update of Medicare Enrollment in HMOs*. Excelsior, MN: Interstudy, 1987.

Iverson, Laura Himes et al. *Improving Health and Long Term Care for the Elderly: An Examination of Medicare Capitation and HMOs*. Excelsior, MN: Interstudy, 1986.

J

Jacobs, Lee D. "The HMO physician." *HMO Practice* 4(6): 203-205. November/December 1990.

Jacobs, Lee. "Making the change: fee-for-service to HMO." *HMO Practice* 4(6): 215-219. November/December 1990.

Joffe, Mark. "Recent developments in hold harmless provisions for managed care organizations." *Medical Interface* 3(7): 44-45, 48. July 1990.

Joffe, Mark and Gold, Marsha. "Trends in health maintenance organization pharmacy benefits and practices." *Drug Benefit Trends* 2(6): 5-9. November-December 1990.

Johnson, J. D. "Proper respect." *HMO Practice* 4(1): 34-5. January-February 1990.

Johnson, Jeanie M. (ed.) *Introduction to Alternative Delivery Mechanisms: HMOs, PPOs, and CMPs.* Washington, DC: National Health Lawyers Associations, 1986.

Johnson, Maryfran. "An IS Approach to managed care." *Computerworld* 25(20): 89, 93. May 20, 1991.

Johnson, Robin E. "Technology assessment." *HMO Practice* 4(5): 181-182. September-October 1990.

Johnsson, J. "EPO helps hospital save millions on employee benefits." *Hospitals* 65(21): 69-70. November 5, 1991.

Johnsson, J. "Forming own PPO helps hospital gain efficiency." *Hospitals* 65(12): 70, 72. June 20, 1991.

Johnsson, Julie. "Case study: managed care helps hospital contain costs." *Hospitals* 65(5): 40-44. March 5, 1991.

Johnsson, Julie. "Developing a winning strategy for managed care contracting." *Hospitals* 65(19): 26-30. October 5, 1991.

Jones, Katherine R. "Feasibility analysis of preferred provider organizations." *Journal of Nursing Administration* 20(1): 28-33. January 1990.

Jones, Michael B. and Beauregard, Thomas R. "HMO cost-control strategies." *Journal of Compensation & Benefits* 7(2): 47-50. September/October 1991.

K

Kalish, Ruth. "Humana tries important entry into Chicago market." *Health Care Strategic Management* 8(11): 11-16. November 1990.

Kanute, Michael. "Evolving theories of malpractice liability for HMOs." *Specialty Law Digest Health Care.*

Kaplan, Jeffrey G. "Managed care is data management." *Physician Executive* 16(4): 20-24. July/August 1990.

Katz, Amy. "HMO profits on upswing despite flat enrollment." *Business Insurance* 25(30): 38-39. July 29, 1991.

Katz, Harvey P. "Quality telephone medicine." *HMO Practice* 4(4): 137-141. July/August 1990.

Katz, Harvey P. *Telephone Medicine Triage and Training: a Handbook for Primary Care Health Professionals.* Thorofare, NJ: SLACK, Inc., 1990.

Katz, Leonard A. "Who is the HMO physician?" *HMO Practice* 4(6): 201-202. November/December 1990.

Keane, Richard M. "The PPO potential." *Best's Review (Prop/Casualty)* 92(3): 49-50, 94. July 1991.

Kelleher, David E. "Should an HMO enter the TPA business?" *Medical Interface* 3(12): 8-10, 12, 37. December 1990.

Kelly, Donald K. "how to Avoid "bed-day tricks" in managed care." *National Underwriter (Property/Casualty/Employee Benefits)* 95(28): 14-15. July 15, 1991.

Kemper, Donald W. "Members are providers, too." *HMO Magazine* 31(6): 6-7. November/December 1990.

Kenkel, Paul J. "Facilities slow to join medicaid HMOs." *Modern Healthcare* 21(25): 32-38. June 24, 1991.

Kenkel, Paul J. "HMOs form networks to serve firms with offices in more than one region." *Modern Healthcare* 21(27): 37-38. July 8, 1991.

Kenkel, Paul J. "HMOs show new signs of consolidation." *Modern Healthcare* 21(23): 50-51. June 10, 1991.

Kenkel, Paul J. "Improving managed care's management." *Modern Healthcare* 20(19): 27-28, 34. May 14, 1990.

Kenkel, Paul J. "Income gain allows HMO to hold premium hike to 11%." *Modern Healthcare* 21(15): 26. April 15, 1991.

Kenkel, Paul J. "Managed-care plans with provider financial backing report growth; about half see profit." *Modern Healthcare* 21(20): 96-102. May 20, 1991.

Kenkel, Paul J. "Managed-care projects strive for affordable long-term care." *Modern Healthcare* 21(2): 41. January 14, 1991.

Kenkel, Paul J. "Managed-care organizations on the rebound." *Modern Healthcare* 20(20): 82, 84-86, 88. May 21, 1990.

Kenkel, Paul J. "More hospitals seek managed-care specialists." *Modern Healthcare* 21(2): 36-37. January 14, 1991.

Kenkel, Paul J. "Program's enrollees learn from leaders." *Modern Healthcare* 20(19): 38, 41. May 14, 1990.

Kenkel, Paul J. "Proposed rule change might sweeten HMOs for employers, speed spread of managed care." *Modern Healthcare* 21(37): 34. September 16, 1991.

Kent, Jim. "The role of employee assistance programs in managed mental health care." *Medical Interface* 3(8): 25-26, 28. August 1990.

Kertesz, Louise. "Digital devises own standards to judge HMO performance." *Business Insurance* 25(33): 16-17. August 19, 1991.

Kertesz, Louise. "Managed care approach." *Business Insurance* 25(37): 3, 18-20. September 16, 1991.

Klitsner, Irving. "The pediatrician in an HMO." *HMO Practice* 4(6): 206-208. November/December 1990.

Knickman, James R. and McCall, Nelda. "A prepaid managed approach to long-term care." *Health Affairs* 4(1): 90-104. Spring 1986.

Koco, Linda. "Competition spurs growth of point-of-service HMOs; point-of-service HMOs will grow like corn." *National Underwriter (Life/Health/Financial Services)* 95(17): 7-9. April 29, 1991.

Koco, Linda. "Point-of-service HMOs are growing rapidly." *National Underwriter (Property/Casualty/Employee Benefits)* 95(23): 15, 17. June 10, 1991.

Koco, Linda. "Studies focus on managed care." *National Underwriter (Life/Health/Financial Services)* 95(16): 19, 27. April 22, 1991.

Kollar, K. M.; Deady, J. E.; and Dillon, M. J. "Comprehensive pharmaceutical services in the outpatient surgery department." *American Journal of Hospital Pharmacy* 47(2): 343-346. February 1990.

Kongstvedt, Peter R. (ed.) *The Managed Health Care Handbook.* Rockville, MD: Aspen Publishers, 1989.

Koocher, Glenn S. "Turning over a new leaf." *HMO Magazine* 31(6): 17-21. November/December 1990.

Korenchuck, Keith M. "Negotiating and analyzing managed care contracts." *Medical Group Management Journal* 38(1): 37-38, 40. January/February 1991.

Kouba, David J. "Primary care providers: managing today's prepaid risk." *Medical Group Management Journal* 38(1): 37-38, 40. January/February 1991.

Kralewski, John E. et al. "Strategies employed by HMOs to achieve hospital discounts: a case study of seven HMOs." *Health Care Management Review* 16(1): 9-16. Winter 1991.

Krasner, Wendy. "HMO-employer contract: an opportunity for a creative partnership." *Group Health Journal* 4(2): 16-23. Summer 1983.

Kraus, Nancy; Porter, Michelle; and Ball, Patricia. *Managed Care: A Decade in Review 1980-1990. A Special Edition of The Interstudy Edge.* Excelsior, MN: InterStudy. July 1991.

Kretz, Sandra; Sommers, Christie; and Aquilina, David. "PPOs: lessons from the '80s, issues for the '90s." *Employer's Health Benefits Bulletin* 4(5): 7-8. June 1990.

Kugelman, Larry. "Choosing Among HMOs." *Business Insurance* 25(23): 29. June 10, 1991.

Kushner, K. P. et al. "Critical incidents in family practice — cases and commentaries." New York: Springer, 1982. (See esp. Chapters 14, 15, 16, 26).

L

Ladden, M. "On-site perinatal case management: an HMO model." *Journal of Perinatal & Neonatal Nursing* 5(1): 27-32. June 1991.

Landgraf, Gerald. "The effectiveness of managed care programs." *Medical Interface* 4(9): 12-13, 22. September 1991.

Langwell, Kathryn M. "Structure and performance of health maintenance organizations: a review." *Health Care Financing Review* 12(1): 71-79. Fall 1990.

Langwell, Kathryn M. and Hadley, James P. "Insights from the Medicare HMO demonstrations." *Health Affairs* 9(1): 74-84. Spring 1990.

Lapham S. C.; Kring, M. K.; and Skipper B. "Prenatal behavioral risk screening by computer in a health maintenance organization-based prenatal care clinic." *American Journal of Obstetrics & Gynecology* 165(3): 506-14. September 1991.

Lapham, Sandra C.; Montgomery, Kelly A.; and Hoy, Wendy E. "HMO databases: fertile ground for epidemiological research." *Computers in Healthcare* 18-20, 22, 24. September 1990.

Lawless, Grant D. "A managed care approach to outpatient substance abuse treatment." *Benefits Quarterly* 6(1): 30-36. First Quarter, 1990.

Lawrence D. M. "A provider's view of prevention approaches in a prepaid group practice." *Cancer* 67(6 Suppl): 1767-71. March 15, 1991.

Lawrence, David. "Learning from HMOs." *Health Management Quarterly* 7(3): 12-15. Third Quarter, 1990.

Leutz, Walter et al. "Financial performance in the social health maintenance organization, 1985-88." *Health Care Financing Review* 12(1): 9-18. Fall 1990.

Leutz, Walter N. et al. *Changing Health Care for an Aging Society.* Lexington, MA: DC Heath/Lexington Books, 1985.

Levin, Rebecca. A. "Hospitals and managed care: a solution to the puzzle." *Medical Interface* 3(8): 37-38, 43-44. August 1990.

Leyland, Arthur, Jr. "Managed care in the 1990s." *Journal of Medical Practice* 6(3): 161-165. Winter 1991.

Lichtenstein R. et al. "Selection bias in TEFRA at-risk HMOs." *Medical Care* 29(4): 318-31. April 1991.

Locke, Adrienne C. "HMOs strong in cities." *Business Insurance* 25(3): 3, 28. January 21, 1991.

Lopez, Lisa. "HMOs go high-tech." *HMO Magazine* 31(4): 12-15, 27, 28-30. July/August 1990.

Lopez, Lisa. "Link me up, Scotty! Could HMO networks be the next wave of managed care?" *HMO Magazine* 32(1): 20-24. January/February 1991.

Lopez, Lisa. "Medical technology assessment: who decides?" *HMO Magazine* 32(2): 20-23, 30-32. March/April 1991.

The Loran Commission: A Report to the Community. Brookline, MA: Harvard Community Health Plan, 1989.

Loucks, Vernon R., Jr. "Managed care from above." *Business & Health* 9(6): 85-87. June 1991.

Louis Harris and Associates, Inc. *A Report Card on HMOs: 1980-1984.* Prepared for the Henry J. Kaiser Family Foundation. New York: Louis Harris & Associates, 1985. (Study No. 844885). *Summary Report* also available.

Luce, Gregory M. and Gustafson, Mark D. "A foot to stand on." *HMO Magazine* 31(5): 25-26. September-October 1990.

Luce, Gregory M. and Gustafson, Mark D. "Managed care liabilities for employers." *Business & Health* 8(9): 66, 68. September 1990.

Luce, Gregory M. and Gustafson, Mark D. "Potential liability when a health plan fails." *Business & Health* 9(2): 70, 71. February 1991.

Luft, Harold S. "Assessing the evidence of HMO performance." *Milbank Memorial Fund Quarterly/Health and Society* 58(4): 501-536. 1980.

Luft, Harold S. "Translating the US HMO experience to other health systems." *Health Affairs* 10(3). Fall 1991.

Luft, Harold S. "Trends in medical care costs: do HMOs lower the rate of growth? *Medical Care* 18(1): 1-16. 1980.

Luft, Harold S. *Health Maintenance Organizations: Dimensions of Performance*. New York: John Wiley & Sons, 1981.

Lurye, Donald R. "Why I love my HMO." *Medical Economics* 68(7): 118, 120, 123-124. April 8, 1991.

Lutz, Sandy. "Managed care widens graduates' job field." *Modern Healthcare* 20(34): 37. August 27, 1990.

Lyon, Ronald A. "Formulary-control procedures in a staff-model health maintenance." *American Journal of Hospital Pharmacy* 47(2): 340-342. February 1990.

M

Mackie, D. L. and Decker, D. K. *Group and IPA HMOs*. Rockville, MD: Aspen Systems Corporation, 1981.

Madlin, Nancy. "EPO: latest beast in the managed care menagerie." *Business & Health* 9(3): 48, 50-53. March 1991.

"Managed care poised to dominate health delivery and financing during this decade." *Managed Care Outlook* 3(6): 1-10. March 16, 1990.

"Managed care to grow, but can be dealt with profitably." *Managed Care Outlook Special Report* 3(8): 1-3, 5-6. April 13, 1990.

Managed Care Under Medicaid: The Need for Change. Detroit, MI: Comprehensive Health Services, Inc. & Wellcorp, Inc., 1990.

Manning, Willard G. et al. "A controlled trial of the effect of a prepaid group practice on use of services." *New England Journal of Medicine* 310(23): 1505-1510. June 7, 1984.

Manning, Willard G. et al. *Use of Outpatient Mental Health Care: Trial of a Prepaid Group Practice Versus Fee-for-Service*. Santa Monica, CA: Rand Corporation, August 1986.

Margo, Katherine L. and Margo, Geoffrey M. "Practical application of a patient satisfaction survey." *HMO Practice* 4(3): 104-108. May/June 1990.

Margolis, Robin Elizabeth. "OBRA '90: preview of nationalized health care?" *HealthSpan* 7(11): 21-26. December 1990.

Marion Laboratories, Inc. *Marion Managed Care Digest: HMO Edition*. Kansas City, MO: Marion Laboratories, May 1989.

Marion Laboratories, Inc. *Marion Managed Care Digest: HMO Pharmacy Edition*. Kansas City, MO: Marion Laboratories, May 1989.

Marion Managed Care Digest — PPO Edition. Kansas City, MO: Marion Laboratories, 1989.

Marion Managed Care Digest Update. Kansas City, MO: Marion Laboratories, 1989.

Marion Managed Care Digest: HMO Edition. Kansas City, MO: Marion Merrell Dow, 1990.

Marion Managed Care Digest: HMO Pharmacy Edition. Kansas City, MO: Marion Laboratories, 1990.

Marion Merrell Dow Managed Care Digest: HMO and HMO Pharmacy Edition. Kansas City, MO: Marion Merrell Dow, 1991.

Marion Merrell Dow Managed Care Digest: PPO edition. Kansas City, MO: Marion Merrell Dow, 1990.

Marion Merrell Dow Managed Care Digest: Update Edition. Kansas City, MO: Marion Merrell Dow, 1990.

Market, Financial and Operating Statistics for HMOs. Gwynedd, PA: Sherlock Company, Summer 1990.

"Market HMO, PPO connections for special competitive edge." *Health Care Competition Week Special Report* 7(36): 1-8. September 10, 1990.

Mascia, Frank R. "Managing through a turnaround." *Medical Interface* 4(4): 40-42, 44. April 1991.

Mayer, T. R. "Family practice referral patterns in a health maintenance organization." *Journal of Family Practice* 14(2): 315-319. 1982.

Mayer, T. R. and Mayer, C. G. *The Health Insurance Alternative: A Complete Guide to Health Maintenance Organizations*. New York: Putnam Publishing Group, 1984.

Mayer, Thomas R. and Mayer, Gloria G. "HMOs: origins and development." *New England Journal of Medicine* 312(9): 590-594. February 28, 1985.

McCabe, Dawn M.; Greenberg, Carol; and Bradbury, Robert C. "Eight steps to discourage adverse selection." *Business & Health* 8(2): 17. February 1990.

McCombs, Jeffrey S.; Kasper, Judith D.; and Riley, Gerald F. "Do HMOs reduce health care costs? A multivariate analysis of two Medicare HMO demonstration projects." *Health Services Research* 25(4): 593-613. October 1990.

McCurren, J. K. "Factors for success: capitated primary physicians in Medicare HMOs." *Health Care Management Review* 16(2): 49-53. Spring 1991.

McDonald, Martha. "Domestic partner benefits changes." *Business & Health* 8(10): 11-12, 14, 16 passim. October 1990.

McDonald, Martha. "The case for managed dental." *HMO Magazine* 31(5): 6-8. September-October 1990.

McEachern, Sharon. "Point-of-service: communication is the key to success." *Business & Health* 9(12): 47-49. November 1991.

McElwee, N. E. et al. "An observational study of isotretinoin recipients treated for acne in a health maintenance organization." *Archives of Dermatology* 127(3): 341-6. March 1991.

McFarnland, Bentson H. *Retention and Use of Services by Severely Mentally Ill HMO Members: Report of a Pilot Study*. Portland, OR: Kaiser Permanente, October 2, 1990.

McGarvey, Michael R. "Physicians and managed care programs." *Bulletin of the New York Academy of Medicine* 66(1): 71-9. January-February 1990.

McGuire, Peggy. "Kaiser Permanente's new technologies committee: an approach to assessing technology." *Quality Review Bulletin* 16(6): 240-242. June 1990.

McManis, G.; Abramowitz, K.; and L. Piccolo. "Three experts, three visions of the future." (Interview by Laura Souhrada.) *Hospitals* 65(7): 41-3. April 5, 1991.

"Measures of success: Interview with Humana Health Care Division President Wayne Smith." *HMO Magazine* 31(6): 9-11. September-October 1990.

Mechanic, D. (ed.) *Handbook of Health, Health Care, and the Health Professions.* New York: Free Press, 1983.

Meier, Gerald B. and Aquilina, David. *Evaluating Health Maintenance Organizations: A Guide for Business, Labor and Coalitions.* Excelsior, MN: Interstudy, 1982.

Menges, Joel J.; Snow, David B. Jr.; and Williamson, Karen E. "Managed care: going public in a new way." *Medical Interface* 4(3): 49-50. March 1991.

Menges, Joel. "Consolidation in the HMO industry: is it for better or for worse?" *Medical Interface* 3(8): 49-50, 53. August 1990.

Menges, Joel. *Evaluating HMO Industry Performance: Lessons From the 1980s, Challenges for the 1990s.* Rockville, MD: American International Healthcare, Inc., 1990.

Metz, Pamela. "The Maryland experience." *HMO Magazine* 32(1): 10-12. January/February 1991.

Michaels, Joel L. *Legal Issues in the Fee-for-Service/Prepaid Medical Group.* (A monograph in the Going Prepaid Series). Denver, CO: Center for Research in Ambulatory Health Care Administration, Medical Group Management Association, 1983.

Miller, Christine. "Are HMOs the answer?" *HMO Practice* 4(5): 183-184. September/October 1990.

Minding America's Mental Health: Trends in Mental Health Coverage. Washington, DC: National Association of Private Psychiatric Hospitals, 1991.

Mitchell, John H. and Dunn, James P. "Employees' choice of a health plan & their subsequent satisfaction." *Journal of Occupational Medicine* 26(5): 361-366. May 1984.

Mollica, Robert L.; Tessler, Julie; and Chung, Thomas. *Coordinating Community Care for Frail Elders in Health Maintenance Organizations.* Boston, MA: Executive Office of Elder Affairs, November 1990.

Moore, Gordon T. "Health maintenance organizations and medical education: breaking the barriers." *Academic Medicine* 65(7): 427-432. July 1990.

Moran, Donald W. and Savela, Theresa E. "HMOs, finance, and the hereafter." *Health Affairs* 5(1): 51-65. Spring 1986.

"More HMO enrollees get choice of care provider." *Modern Healthcare* 20(16): 33. April 23, 1990.

Morrison, Ellen M. and Luft, Harold S. "Health maintenance organization environments in the 1980s and beyond." *Health Care Financing Review* 12(1): 81-90. Fall 1990.

Mulcahy, Colleen. "Exposure in managed care seen." *National Underwriter (Property/Casualty/Employee Benefits)* 95(16): 9, 16. April 22, 1991.

Mulcahy, Colleen. "High-flying HMO stocks seen headed for earth." *National Underwriter (Life/Health/Financial Services)* 95(13): 4, 49. April 1, 1991.

Mulcahy, Colleen. "Lincoln Nat'l opts out of managed care market." *National Underwriter (Life/Health/Financial Services)* 95(39): 3, 5. September 30, 1991.

Mulcahy, Colleen. "Managed care assumptions 'untested, unproven'." *National Underwriter (Life/Health/Financial Services)* 95(18): 51, 55. May 6, 1991.

Mulcahy, Colleen. "PPOs facing period of consolidation." *National Underwriter (Life/Health/Financial Services)* 95(8): 3, 8. February 25, 1991.

Murphy, G. "Quality assurance in outpatient medical records." *Topics in Health Records Management* 10(3): 59-69. March 1990.

N

Nash, D. *Future Practice Alternatives in Medicine.* New York: Igaku-Shoin, 1987.

National Managed Care Firms 1990. Excelsior, MN: InterStudy, 1990.

"National trends in health benefits cost containment strategies." *Federation of American Health Systems Review* 23(6): 38-9. November-December 1990.

Neal, Patricia A. *Management Information Systems for the Fee-For-Service/Prepaid Medical Group.* (A monograph in the Going Prepaid Series). Denver, CO: Center for Research in Ambulatory Health Care Administration, Medical Group Management Association, 1983.

Nelson, Carl W. and Niederberger, Jane. "Patient satisfaction surveys: an opportunity for total quality improvement." *Hospital & Health Services Administration* 35(3): 409-427. Fall 1990.

Nelson, Lyle et al. "Medigap preferred provider organizations: issues, implications, and early experience." *Health Care Financing Review* 12(4): 87-97. Summer 1991.

Nemes, Judith. "Humana asks Ky. for HMO exemption." *Modern Healthcare* 20(19): 2. May 14, 1990.

Nemes, Judith. "Humana to buy Chicago Hospital, HMO." *Modern Healthcare* 20(40): 3-4. October 8, 1990.

Nemes, Judith. "Humana won't need CON for Michael Reese." *Modern Healthcare* 20(45): 4. November 12, 1990.

Newcomer, R.; Harrington, C.; and Friedlob, A. "Awareness and enrollment in the Social/HMO." *Gerontologist* 30(1): 86-93. February 1990.

Newcomer, Robert; Harrington, Charlene; and Friedlob, Alan. "Social health maintenance organizations: assessing their initial experiences." *Health Services Research* 25(3): 425-454. August 1990.

The 1983 Investors Guide to Health Maintenance Organizations. Washington, DC Government Printing Office, 1983. (GPO Stock #017-002-001585-5).

1989 Managed Care Executive Compensation Survey. Montara, CA: J. Richards & Co., January 1989.

"The 1990 national executive poll on health care costs and benefits." *Business & Health* 8(4): 25-26, passim. April 1990.

"1990s will bring continued maturation of the managed care industry." *Managed Care Outlook* 3(5): 1-4. March 2, 1990.

Nirtaut, Dennis J. "Ask a benefits manager: make data meaningful to analyze health costs." *Business Insurance* 25(19): 49. May 13, 1991.

Noda, B. and Austin, N. "How Pacific Telesis put health care costs on hold." *Business & Health* 8(11): 52, 54-6. November 1990.

Norquist, G. S. and Wells, K. B. "How do HMOs reduce outpatient mental health care costs?" *American Journal of Psychiatry* 148(1): 96-101. January 1991.

O

O'Connor, Kathleen. "Employers and managed care; risky business: HMOs and managed care." *Business & Health* 9(6): 8-9, 30-34. June 1991.

Oberg, Charles N. and Longseth-Polich, Cynthia. *Medicaid-Entering the Third Decade: Enrollment in HMOs and Alternative Health Systems.* Excelsior, MN: Interstudy, 1986.

Ogden, David F. "The dynamics of managed care underwriting." *Medical Interface* 4(2): 50-51, 58. February 1991.

Oliver, Richard C. et al. "Dentist participation in health maintenance organizations. A case study." *Journal of the American College of Dentistry* 57(2): 9-13. Summer 1990.

Orland, Burton I. "Prescription mailing service for seniors." *HMO Practice* 4(3): 102-3. May-June 1990.

Otis, L. H. "Brokers view managed care as key in WC." *National Underwriter (Property/Casualty/Employee Benefits)* 95(46): 11, 60. November 18, 1991.

Ottensmeyer, D. J. and Key M. K. "Lessons learned hiring HMO medical directors." *Health Care Management Review* 16(2): 21-30. Spring 1991.

P

Pacione, Anthony. "A return on investment." *HMO Magazine* 31(3): 16-18. May/June 1990.

Pallarito, Karen. "Public service junkie: Drew E. Altman." *Modern Healthcare* 20(35): 48. September 3, 1990.

Palmer, H. R. et al. "A randomized controlled trial of quality assurance in sixteen ambulatory care practices." *Medical Care* 23: 751-770. 1985.

Palsbo, Susan J. and Gold, Marsha Ruth. HMO Industry Profile: Volume 3: Financial Performance, 1988. Washington, DC: GHAA, June 1990.

Palsbo, Susan J. and Gold, Marsha Ruth. *HMO Industry Profile: Volume 3: Financial Performance, 1989.* Washington, DC: GHAA, June 1990.

Palsbo, Susan J. *HMO Market Penetration in the 30 Largest Metropolitan Statistical Areas, 1989.* Washington, DC: GHAA, December 1990.

Palsbo, Susan Jelley. *Medicare Capitation Explained.* Washington, DC: GHAA, March 1990.

Patricelli, Robert, "Musings of a blind man — reflections on the health care industry." *Health Affairs* 5(2): 128-134. Summer 1986.

Patterson, Daniel Y. "Managed care: an approach to rational psychiatric treatment." *Hospital and Community Psychiatry* 41(10): 1092-5. October 1990.

Pauly, Mark V.; Hillman, Alan L.; and Kerstein, Joseph. "Managing physician incentives in managed care: the role of for-profit ownership." *Medical Care* 28(11): 1013-1024. November 1990.

Peril and Perplexity in HMO Pricing: A Case Study. Spring House, PA: Health Economics, Inc., 1990.

Perry, Linda. "Henry Ford derives profits from diversity." *Modern Healthcare* 20(50): 33-5, 38. December 17, 1990.

Peterson-More, Diana L. "How we built our PPO." *Business & Health* Special Issue, 15-17. 1990.

Pfizer National Healthcare Operations. *How Benefit Managers Choose Health Plans: A National Survey.* New York: Pfizer Pharmaceutical Group, 1990.

Philbin, Patricia and Altman, Diane. "HIV/AIDS home care: an HMO experience." *Caring* 9(8): 42-43, 45. August 1990.

Pickens, Judy E. "Group health options showing potential of market-responsive HMO/indemnity hybrid." *Healthcare Marketing Report* 9(5): 8-10. May 1991.

Polich, Cynthia et al. "The provision of home health services through health maintenance organizations: the role of the physician." *Quality Review Bulletin* 16(5): 170-181. May 1990.

Porell, Frank W. and Turner, Winston M. "Biased selection under an experimental enrollment and marketing Medicare HMO broker." *Medical Care* 28(7): 604-615. July 1990.

Porell, Frank W. and Turner, Winston M. "Biased selection under the senior health plan prior use capitation formula." *Inquiry* 27(1): 39-50. Spring 1990.

Porell, Frank W. and Wallack, Stanley S. "Medicare risk contracting: determinants of market entry." *Health Care Financing Review* 12(2): 75-85. Winter 1990.

Porell, Frank W.; Tompkins, Christopher P.; and Turner, Winston M. "Alternative geographic configurations for Medicare payments to health maintenance organizations." *Health Care Financing Review* 11(3): 17-30. Spring 1990.

Potter, John W. "Understanding utilization data and detecting provider gaming." *Topics in Health Care Financing* 16(3): 28-35. Spring 1990.

Prescott, Richmond. "HMOs and AIDS." *HMO Practice* 4(4): 117-118. July/August 1990.

Preston, J. A. and Retchin, S. M. "The management of geriatric hypertension in health maintenance organizations." *Journal of the American Geriatrics Society* 39(7): 683-90. July 1991.

Puelz, Robert. "A selection model for employees confronted with health insurance alternatives." *Benefits Quarterly* 7(2): 18-22. Second Quarter 1991.

Q

Quinn, Richard D. "Managed care defined - and dissected." *Employer's Health Benefits Bulletin* 4(5): 4-5. June 1990.

Quirk, Michael P.; Truscott, Al; and Stuart Michael. "Managed care personalities." *Group Practice Journal* 39(4): 66, 68-72. July/August 1990.

R

Rader, P. J. "Back to the basics." *HMO Magazine* 31(4): 16-19. July/August 1990.

Rader, P. J. "The mental health package." *HMO Magazine* 31(6): 12-16, 28. November/December 1990.

Randall, Deborah A. "Legal issues in home health affecting managed care in the 1990s." *Medical Interface* 3(11): 32-33, 37-38. November 1990.

Reece, Richard L. and Coombes, David H. "Minnesota's fifteen-year romance." *Group Practice Journal* 39(4): 18, 20-22, 24. July/August 1990.

Regan, John, III; Stanger, Janice; and Powers, Patricia. "Measuring employee satisfaction." *Business & Health* 9(12): 78, 80. November 1991.

Reis, Janet. "Medicaid maternal and child health care: Prepaid plans vs. private fee-for-service." *Research in Nursing and Health* 13(3): 163-71. June 1990.

Retchin, S. M. and Brown B. "Elderly patients with congestive heart failure under prepaid care." *American Journal of Medicine* 90(2): 236-42. February 1991.

Rice, Faye. "America's hottest HMO." *Fortune* 124(2): 94. July 15, 1991.

Richardson, Karen. *HMO Buyer's Guide*. Atlanta, GA: Healthplan Management Services (HPMS), 1991.

Richardson, Kristin M. "How do physician assistants practice in your HMO?" *HMO Practice* 4(5): 167-168. September-October 1990.

Riley, G.; Lubitz, J.; and Rabey, E. "Enrollee health status under Medicare risk contracts: an analysis of mortality rates." *Health Services Research* 26(2): 137-63. June 1991.

Riley, Trish and Coburn, Andrew F. *Medicaid Managed Care: The State of the Art. A Guide for States*. Portland, Maine: National Academy for State Health Policy, September 1990.

Robinson, J. C. et al. "A method for risk-adjusting employer contributions to competing health insurance plans." *Inquiry* 28(2): 107-16. Summer 1991.

Rockman, Scott I. 1991 *HMO/PPO Directory*. Stanford, CT: Medical Device Register, 1991.

Rolph, Elizabeth S. "Introducing the preferred provider organization option into health benefit plans: Three case studies." Elizabeth S. Rolph, supported by the US Department of Health and Human Services. Santa Monica, CA: RAND Corporation, 1990.

Ross, Donna J. and Hughes, Kathleen E. "A new attitude: contracting for success with alternative delivery systems." *Journal of Ambulatory Care Management* 10(1): 1-21. 1987.

Rossiter, Louis F. and Adamache, Killard W. "Payment to health maintenance organizations and the geographic factor." *Health Care Financing Review* 12(1): 19-30. Fall 1990.

Roth, Michael D. "Legal Consideration for Utilization Management." *Utilization Review: The Key to Managed Health Care Delivery*. Section 6. San Francisco, California, July 31-August 2, 1986. Washington, DC GHAA, 1986.

"Routing seniors into HMOs: Medicare is losing ground." *HealthSpan* 7(7): 14-16. July/August 1990.

Rymer, T. A. "HMO liable for the negligence of a non-HMO consulting physician." *Indiana Medicine* 83(2): 130-1. February 1990.

S

Sabin, J. E. "Clinical skills for the 1990s: six lessons from HMO practice." *Hospital & Community Psychiatry* 42(6): 605-8. June 1991.

Sales & Marketing Management Resources. *1990/91 Managed Care Marketing, Sales, and Support/Service Practices Study*. Montara, CA: J. Richard & Co., 1991.

Savitz, Eric J. "No miracle cure: HMOs are not the rx for spiraling health-care costs." *Barron's* 71(31): 8-9, 21-23. August 5, 1991.

Saxl, Linda R. "Keeping up with changes in managed health care programs." *Employee Benefits Digest* 27(3): 1, 7-8, 10, 12. March 1990.

Schachner, Michael. "Firms drop HMOs to increase bargaining power." *Business Insurance* 25(7): 78-79. February 18, 1991.

Schachner, Michael. "Study finds gains in workers' rating of managed care." *Business Insurance* 25(44): 1, 111. November 4, 1991.

Schafer, Eldon and Gocke, Michael E. *Management Accounting for Health Maintenance Organizations*. Denver, CO: Center for Research in Ambulatory Health Care Administration, an affiliate of the Medical Group Management Association, 1984.

Schafer, Eldon L.; Zulauf, Dwight J.; and Gocke, Michael E. *Management Accounting for Fee-for-Service/Prepaid Medical Groups*. Denver, CO: Center for Research in Ambulatory Health Care Administration, an affiliate of the Medical Group Management Association, 1985.

Schafer, Eldon et al. *Evaluating the Performance of a Prepaid Medical Group: A Management Audit Manual*. (A monograph in the Going Prepaid Series.) Denver, CO: Center for Research in Ambulatory Health Care Administration, Medical Group Management Association, 1985.

Schaller, Donald F. "The seven components of an HMO - an overview." *Management and Physician Orientation Program*. Section 2. Los Angeles, California, March 19-21, 1987. Washington, DC: GHAA, 1987.

Scheur, Barry S. and Stone, Diane L. *An HMO Regulatory Primer*. Newton Center, MA: NAHMOR Educational Foundation, April 1988.

Scheur, Barry S. and Stone, Diane L. *An HMO Regulatory Primer.* Newton Center, MA: Scheur Management Group & Nat'l Assn of HMO Reg Ed Found, 1989.

Schlesinger, Mark et al. "Profits under pressure: the economic performance of investor-owned and nonprofit health maintenance organizations." *Medical Care* 24(7): 615-627. July 1986.

Schmidt, John J. *Tricks of the Trade.* Spring House, PA: Health Economics, 1990.

Schneller, Eugene S. "The leadership and executive potential of physicians in an era of managed care systems." *Hospital & Health Services Administration* 36(1): 43-55. Spring 1991.

Schoenbaum, Stephen C. "Implementation of preventive services in an HMO practice." *Journal of General Internal Medicine* 5(5 Suppl): S123-S127. September-October 1990.

Schorr, Alvin L. "Health care in America: what's new? what's next?" *Management Quarterly* 32(2): 33-37. Summer 1991.

Schryver, Darrell L. "Responding to managed care proposals." *Medical Group Management Journal* 38(1): 32-34. January/February 1991.

Schuch, Rick J. et al. "A student health HMO as a partnership model within an academic medical center." *Journal of Family Practice* 30(5): 585-91. May 1990.

Schulman, Kevin M. and Lynn, Lorna A. "A primer on cost-effectiveness studies." *Drug Benefit Trends* 2(3): 13-14, 16-17. May/June 1990.

Schultz, P. R. "Health access report. Managed care." *Washington Nurse* 21(5): 16-7. June 1991.

Schulz, Rockwell et al. "Physician adaptation to health maintenance organizations and implications for management." *Health Services Research* 25[1(partl)]: 43-64. April 1990.

Schwartz, Dan and Lopez, Lisa. "Measuring up." *HMO Magazine* 31(3): 12-14. May/June 1990.

Schwartz, Matthew. "HMO plan automates health delivery process." *National Underwriter (Life/Health/Financial Services)* 95(28): 12-13. July 15, 1991.

Scott, Malvise A. "Prepayment and CHCs in North Carolina." *Journal of Ambulatory Care Management* 13(4): 41-45. October 1990.

Sedere, Lloyd I. and St. Clair, R. Lawrence. "Quality assurance and managed mental health care." *Psychiatric Clinics of North America* 13(1): 89-97. March 1990.

Shadle, Maureen; Gruber, Lynn R.; and Hunter, Mary M. *1989 National Managed Care Firms.* Excelsior, MN: InterStudy and Center for Managed Care Research, December 1989.

Shapiro, Sam "Review of Twenty Years of Research on HMOs." *HMO Data Management: Demands and Responses.* Section 10. Minneapolis, Minnesota, November 3-5, 1985. Washington, DC: GHAA, 1985.

Sharp, William T. and Strandberg, Lee R. "Contracting by managed care systems for pharmaceutical products an services." *Topics in Hospital Pharmacy Management* 10(3): 8-17. November 1990.

Sheehan, Thomas P. "The family practitioner in the HMO." *HMO Practice* 4(6): 209-210. November/December 1990.

Sheldon, Alan. *Getting There: A Strategic Planning Framework For Health Maintenance Organizations.* Washington, DC: US DHHS, August 1984.

Shikles, Janet L. *Medicare: GAO Views on Medicare Payments to Health Maintenance Organizations.* Washington, DC: GAO. May 9, 1990. GAO/t-HRD-90-27.

Shouldice, Robert G. "HMO facts and fictions." *Medical Group Management Journal* 37(2): 16, 68. March/April 1990.

Shouldice, Robert G. "HMOs: four models profiled." *Journal of Medical Group Management Association.* 33(3): 8, 9, 33. May/June 1986.

Shouldice, Robert G. *Introduction to Managed Care: Health Maintenance Organizations, Preferred Provider Organizations, and Competitive Medical Plans.* Arlington, VA: Information Resources Press, 1991.

Shouldice, Robert G. *Managed Care: HMOs, PPOs and CMPs.* Arlington, VA: Information Resources Press.

Shouldice, Robert G. *Marketing Management in the Fee-For-Service/Prepaid Medical Group.* (A monograph in the *Going Prepaid* Series.) Denver, CO: Center for Research in Ambulatory Health Care Administration, Medical Group Management Association, 1983.

Siddharthan, Kris. "HMO enrollment by Medicare beneficiaries in heterogeneous communities." *Medical Care* 29(10): 918-927. October 1990.

Silversin, Jack. "The HMO physician as team player." *HMO Practice* 4(6): 226-230. November/December 1990.

Simpson, Rory. "Managed care is more than cost containment." *Business & Health* Supplement, 8-9. 1991.

Singer, Charles J. *Managed Care: Information Systems Vendors.* Marblehead, MA: Charles J. Singer, 1987.

Siu, Albert L. et al. "A fair approach to comparing quality of care." *Health Affairs* 10(1): 62-75. Spring 1991.

Sloss, Elizabeth et al. *Effect of a Health Maintenance Organization of Physiologic Health: Results from a Randomized Trial.* Santa Monica, CA: Rand Corporation, 1987.

Snook, I. Donald and Kaye, Edita M. *A Guide to Health Care Joint Ventures.* Rockville, MD: Aspen Publishers, 1987.

The Social/Health Maintenance Organization: The First Five Years. Social/HMO Consortium, 1990.

Sovner, Robert; Bailey, Katharine P.; and Weisblatt, Richard E. "An HMO psychopharmacology service." *HMO Practice* 4(5): 162-166. September/October 1990.

Sperling, Kenneth L. "Flexible benefits and managed care: making it work." *Benefits Quarterly* 7(2): 6-12. Second Quarter 1991.

Spillane, Janice. "PPO gaining wide acceptance in care plans." *Pension World* 27(5): 18, 20. May 1991.

Standardized HMO Data Form Task Force. *Data Collection Forms.* Washington, DC: GHAA, 1990.

Starr, P. *The Social Transformation of American Medicine.* New York: Basic Books, 1982.

State Anti-Managed Care Legislation: Employer Concerns and Issues. Washington, DC: Washington Business Group on Health, January 1991.

Stein, Gary F. and Kemper, Ronald J. "Health clubs and HMOs." *HMO Practice* 5(1): 7-8. January/February 1991.

Stevens, Carol. "An industry that's booming in spite of itself." *Medical Economics* 68(8): 47-50, 52-53. April 22, 1991.

STFM Task Force on Managed Health Care. Edited by Robert Eidus and Samuel W. Warburton. *Managed Health Care: a Teaching Syllabus.* Society of Teachers of Family Medicine, 1990.

Stimmel, B. "The study and practice of medicine in the twenty-first century: ask not for whom the bell tolls." *Mount Sinai Journal of Medicine* 57(1): 11-24. January 1990.

Stratton, W. T. "Third-party payers and the physician's duty of confidentiality." *Kansas Medicine* 92(4): 92, 111-2. April 1991.

Sullivan, C. B. and Rice T. "The health insurance picture in 1990." *Health Affairs* 10(2): 104-15. Summer 1991.

Survey Findings: Managed Care Initiatives. Lincolnshire, IL: Hewitt Associates, 1991.

Sutton, Harry Jr. and Sorbo, Allen J. *Actuarial Issues in the Fee-For-Service/Prepaid Medical Group.* (A monograph in the *Going Prepaid* Series.) Denver, CO: Center for Research in Ambulatory Health Care Administration, Medical Group Management Association, 1983.

Sutton, Harry L. Jr. and Sorbo, Allen J. *Actuarial Issues in the Fee-for-Service/Prepaid Medical Group.* (*Going Prepaid* Series.) Denver, CO: Center for Research in Ambulatory Health Care Administration, an affiliate of the Medical Group Management Association, 1986.

Sweeney, Robert E. and Rakowski, James P. "Logistical considerations in the prepaid health industry: an exploratory analysis." *Health Marketing Quarterly* 2(2/3): 115-133. Winter/Spring 1985.

Syiek, Joseph A. "Managed care: strategies to help attain future goals." *Medical Interface* 3(7): 31-32, 34, 36. July 1990.

T

T. A. Miller Company and Holland Holland Lynch, Inc., *Attitudes of Physicians with HMO Experience Toward Managed Healthcare.* Kansas City, MO: Marion Laboratories, 1989.

Taravella, Steve. "UniHealth in fast lane after making merge." *Modern Healthcare* 20(23): 59-60, 62, 64-65. June 11, 1990.

Teichman, R. F. and Brandt-Rauf, P. "The need for occupational health nurses in nonindustrial settings." *AAOHN Journal* 38(2): 67-72. February 1990.

Temkin-Greener, H. and Winchell, M. "Medicaid beneficiaries under managed care: provider choice and satisfaction." *Health Services Research* 26(4): 509-29. October 1991.

Terry, Paul E. and Pheley, Alfred M. "Health risks and educational interests in an HMO." *HMO Practice* 5(1): 3-6. January/February 1991.

Thomas, Cynthia and Kelman, Howard R. "Patterns of stability and change in health use among elderly people. Do service systems leave an imprint on behavior?" *Journal of Aging and Health* 3(1): 87-106. February 1991.

Thompson, A. and Rao, C. P. "Who is likely to join a prepaid health care plan? A behavioral approach to identification." *Journal of Health Care Marketing* 10(1): 16-25. March 1990.

Thompson, Roger. "10 ways to cut you health-care cost now." *Nation's Business* 20-23, 26-29. October 1990.

Tokarski, Cathy. "HMO review to switch to random samples." *Modern Healthcare* 21(7): 14. February 18, 1991.

"Top 25 HMOs nationwide ranked by enrollment." HealthWeek 4(4): 34. February 26, 1990.

Topping, Sharon and Fottler, Myron D. "Improved stakeholder management: the key revitalizing the HMO movement?" *Medical Care Review* 47(3): 365-393. Fall 1990.

Traska, Maria R. "Allied-Signal's bold move: is it working?" *Business & Health* 8(4): 18, 20, 23. April 1990.

Traska, Maria R. "Defining managed care." *HMO Magazine* 32(1): 16-19, 30-31. January/February 1991.

Traska, Maria R. "HMO review: will it test whether employers care about quality?" *Business & Health* 8(6): 20, 22, 24, 26, 28, 38. June 1990.

Traska, Maria R. "Self-insurance: can you conquer the risks?" *Business & Health Special Issue,* 10-25. 1990.

Traska, Maria R. "Sign of the times: help wanted." *HMO Magazine* 32(2): 13-18. March/April 1991.

Traska, Maria. "A forgotten link." *HMO Magazine* 31(3): 19-22. May/June 1990.

Trollman, Stephen; Schoopper, Doris; and Torres, Alberto. "Health maintenance organizations in developing countries: what can we expect?" *Health Policy and Planning* 5(2): 149-60. 1990.

U

US Congress, House Select Committee on Aging. "Maintaining Medicare HMO'S : Problems, Protections, and Prospects." Hearing before the Select Committee on Aging, House of Representatives, One hundredth Congress, first session, June 11, 1987. Washington, DC

US Congress. Congressional Budget Office. *Managed Care and the Medicare Program: Background and Evidence.* Washington, DC: May 1990.

US Department of Health and Human Services. *Considerations in Developing a Rural HMO.* Prepared by Interstudy under contract. Washington, DC US DHHS, OHMO, 1985. Part II of a Two-Part series.

US Department of Health and Human Services. *Guide for Fee-For-Service Medical Groups on Affiliation with HMOs.* Technical Assistance Monograph, prepared by Jurgovan and Blair. Washington, DC: US DHHS, OHMO, 1983.

US Department of Health and Human Services. *Guide to Development of Health Maintenance Organizations.* Prepared by Birch and Davis. Washington, DC US DHHS, OHMO, 1982. (GPO Stock #017-002-00154-2).

US Department of Health and Human Services. *Hospitals and HMOs: An Overview of Hospital Sponsorship of Health Maintenance Organizations.* Prepared by Triton Corporation. Washington, DC US DHHS, OHMO, 1982. (DHHS Publication No. (PHS)82-50181).

US Department of Health and Human Services. Bureau of Health Care Delivery and Assistance. *Prepaid Medicaid Chartbook: Selected Enrollment and Utilization Data.* Washington, DC: US DHHS, 1990.

US Deptartment of Health and Human Services. Health Care Financing Administration. *Biased Selection in the TEFRA HMO/CMP Program: Final Report.* Baltimore, MD: HCFA, September 21, 1990.

US Deptartment of Health and Human Services. Health Care Financing Administration. *1991 Adjusted Average Per Capita Cost (AAPCCs) for Tax Equity and Fiscal Responsibility Act of 1982 (TEFRA) Risk Contractors — Information.* Baltimore, MD: HCFA, September 1990.

US Deptartment of Health and Human Services. Office of the Secretary. *Incentive Arrangements Offered by Health Maintenance Organizations and Competitive Medical Plans to Physicians. Volume II.* Washington, DC: DHHS, 1990.

US Deptartment of Health and Human Services. Office of the Secretary. *Incentive Arrangements Offered by Health Maintenance Organizations and Competitive Medical Plans to Physicians. Volume I.* Washington, DC: DHHS, 1990.

US Deptartment of Health and Human Services. Office of Prepaid Health Care. *A Managed Care Model for the Military Departments.* By Douglas A. Braendel. Springfield, VA: National Technical Information Service, May 1990.

US General Accounting Office. *Medicaid: Oversight of Health Maintenance Organizations in the Chicago Area.* Washington, DC: GAO, August 1990. GAO/HRD-90-81.

US General Accounting Office. *Medicare: Second Status Report on Medicare Insured Group Demonstration Projects.* Washington, DC: GAO, June 1990. GAO/HRD-90-117.

US Office of Personnel Management. *1991 FEHBP Premiums.* Washington, DC: OPM, September 1990.

Udvarhelyi, I. S. et al. "Comparison of the quality of ambulatory care for fee-for-service and prepaid patients." *Annals of Internal Medicine* 115(5): 394-400. September 1, 1991.

Ullmann, Ed. "Pains and gains." *HMO Magazine* 31(5): 21-22. September-October 1990.

V

Van Steenwyk, John. *Rate-setting Guidelines for Health Maintenance Organizations.* Spring House, PA: Health Economics, 1989.

Veit, Howard. "Building a bridge to managed care." *Best's Review (Life/Health)* 92(6): 40-44, 146. October 1991.

Vodoor, Mohan. "Logical steps ot successful computerization of pharmacy operations." *Drug Benefit Trends* 1(5): 5, 7-10. November/December 1990.

Von Sternberg, Tom. "Case management for the elderly: benefits for the physician." *HMO Practice* 5(1): 16-18. January/February 1991.

W

Wachsman, Barbara E. and Agnew, Mark W. "HMOs: prospects for the 1990s." *Pension World* 27(7): 41-43. July 1991.

Wadsworth, Peter A. *HMO Investor's Handbook and Securities Pricing Guide.* New York: Wadsworth Company, 1991.

Wagner, E. and Hackenberg, V. *A Practical Guide to Physician Sponsored HMO Development.* Washington, DC: American Society of Internal Medicine, 1986.

Wagner, Lynn. "Medicare managed-care proposal faces skepticism it can cut costs, lure consumers." *Modern Healthcare* 21(28): 32-33. July 15, 1991.

Wagner, Lynn. "Proposal to reduce peer review in HMOs elicits cheers, caution." *Modern Healthcare* 20(23): 36. June 11, 1990.

Ward, Russell A. "Age and patterns of HMO satisfaction." *Journal of Aging and Health* 2(2): 242-260. May 1990.

Ware, John E. et al. "Comparison of health outcomes at a health maintenance organization with those of fee-for-service care (Rand Study)." *Lancet.* May 3, 1986.

Warshaw, Leon J.; Monaghan, John; and Trombly, Preston A. *Employers' Guide to HMOs.* New York: New York Business Group on Health, 1987.

Wasman, J. Mark. "The HMO-IPA relationship: when the time comes to sever the cord." *Medical Interface* 3(9): 41-42, 44. September 1990.

Weimer, Sanford R. "The benefits and drawbacks of managed care." *Hospital and Community Psychiatry* 41(10): 1055. October 1990.

Weiner, J. P. et al. "Impact of managed care on prescription drug use." *Health Affairs* 10(1): 140-54. Spring 1991.

Weiner, Jonathan P. and Ferriss, David M. "GP budget holding in the United Kingdom: learning from American HMOs." *Health Policy* 16(3): 209-20. December 1990.

Weinstein, Robert J. "How to Evaluate the Quality of HMOs." *Journal of Compensation & Benefits* 6(5): 16-19. March/April 1991.

Weiss B. D. and Gardner, C. L. "Consultant utilization by family physicians in a university hospital practice." *Journal of Family Practice* 24(3): 283-285. 1987.

Weiss, Barry D. and Senf, Janet H. "Patient satisfaction survey instrument for use in health maintenance organizations." *Medical Care* 29(5): 434-445. May 1990.

Welch, W. P. "Defining geographic areas to adjust payments to physicians, hospitals, and HMOs." *Inquiry* 28(2): 151-60. Summer 1991.

Welch, W. P. "Health care utilization in HMOs: results from two national samples." *Journal of Health Economics* 4(4): 293-308. December 1985.

Welch, W. P. "The elasticity of demand for health maintenance organizations." *Journal of Human Resources* 21(2): 252-266. Spring 1986.

Welch, W. P. and Frank, R. G. "The predictors of HMO enrollee populations: results from a national sample." *Inquiry* 23(1): 16-22. Spring 1986.

Welch, W. Pete. "Giving physicians incentives to contain costs under Medicaid." *Health Care Financing Review* 12(2): 103-112. Winter 1990

Welch, W. Pete. *HMO Market Share and Its Effect on Local Medicare Costs.* Washington, DC: Urban Institute, March 1991.

Welch, W. Pete; Hillman, Alan L.; and Pauley, Mark V. "Toward new typologies for HMOs." *Milbank Quarterly* 68(2): 221-243. 1990.

Welch, W. Pete; Hillman, Alan L.; and Pauly, Mark V. *Toward a Typology of HMOs Reflecting Financial Incentives to Physicians.* Washington, DC: Urban Institute, October 1989.

Wells, K. B.; Marquis M. S.; and Hosek S. D. "Mental health and selection of preferred providers. Experience in three employee groups." *Medical Care* 29(9): 911-24. September 1991.

Wells, Kenneth B.; Manning, Willard G., Jr.; and Valdez, R. Burciaga. "The effects of a prepaid group practice on mental health outcomes." *Health Services Research* 25(4): 615-625. October 1990.

Weyrauch, Karl F.; Boiko, Patricia E.; and Alvin, Barbara. "Patient sex role and preference for a male or female physician." *Journal of Family Practice* 30(5): 559-562. May 1990.

"What you'd make if you worked for an HMO." *Medical Economics* 7(18): 196. September 17, 1990.

Wilensky, Gail R. and Rossiter, Louis F. "Coordinated care and public programs." *Health Affairs* 10(4): 62-77. Winter 1991.

Wilkinson, P. "Aspects of quality assurance and the link with medical education in the United States." *Postgraduate Medical Journal* 67(784): 176-8. February 1991.

Wittgen, J. S. "HMO contracting presents SNFs with benefits, opportunities." *Provider* 16(4): 20-1. April 1990.

Wojcik, Joanne and Woolsey, Christine. "Growth of traditional HMOs slows: plans go open-ended: Interstudy; firms seeking PPOs, new options: Hewitt." *Business Insurance* 25(10): 3, 10-11, 28. March 11, 1991.

Wojcik, Joanne. "Curbs on managed care hike health costs: study." *Business Insurance* 25(33): 3, 18-19. August 19, 1991.

Wojcik, Joanne. "HMO market: firms bigger, more flexible." *Business Insurance* 24(54): 1, 3-4. December 1990.

Wolfe, Elliott. "Recapturing the flag: restoring the internal medicine residency to its former glory." *HMO Practice* 5(1): 19-21. January/February 1991.

Wood, Steve D. "Service orientation in HMOs." *HMO Practice* 5(2): 35-36. March/April 1991.

Woolsey, Christine. "Accreditation standards for HMOs winning praise." *Business Insurance* 25(32): 2, 74. August 12, 1991.

Woolsey, Christine. "Communication key to managed care plans." *Business Insurance* 25(16): 23. April 22, 1991.

Woolsey, Christine. "Health insurance market: premium increases show no signs of slowing at midyear." *Business Insurance* 25(25): 3-6, 10. June 24, 1991.

Wrightson, Charles William Jr. *HMO Rate Setting & Financial Strategy.* Chicago: Health Administration Press, 1990.

Y

Yox, Susan B. et al. "How does your HMO handle the seasonal demand for school and camp physicals?" *HMO Practice* 4(1): 17-18. January/February 1990.

Z

Zimmerman, Michael. "Medicare: management of the risk-based HMO program," statement of Michael Zimmerman, Senior Associate Director, Human Resources Division, before the Subcommittee on Health, Committee on Ways and Means, House of Representatives. US General Accounting Office, 1988.

Zuvekas, Ann et al. *HMO Outpatient Pharmacy Trends.* Washington DC: Pharmaceutical Manufacturers Association, January 1986.

Zwanziger, J. and Auerbach, R. R. "Evaluating PPO performance using prior expenditure data." *Medical Care* 29(2): 142-51, February 1991.

Glossary

A

Access: An individual's ability to obtain medical services on a timely and financially acceptable basis.

Actuarial: Having to do with probabilities. Actuarial studies performed for HMOs normally consist of projections of utilization and costs of specific benefits for a defined population.

Actuary: An accredited, professionally trained person in insurance mathematics, who calculates rates, reserves, dividends, and other valuations and also makes statistical studies and reports.

Administrative Loading: Or retention as in insurance. The amount added to the prospective actuarial cost of the health care services (pure premium) for expenses of administration, marketing, and profit.

Administrative Services Only (ASO): The providing of such services as: actuarial, benefit plan design, claim processing, data recovery and analysis, employee benefits communication, financial advice, medical care conversions, preparation of data for reports to governmental units, stop-loss coverage, and so on, to a self-insured plan. These services are provided on a contract basis by an insurer or its subsidiary.

Adverse Selection: The phenomenon of the enrollment of a disproportionate percentage of persons who are poorer risks — that is, persons who are more ill, more prone to suffer loss, or to make claims — than the average person.

Anniversary: The beginning of a subscriber group's benefit year. A subscriber group with a year coinciding with the calendar year would be said to have a January 1st anniversary.

Assignment: The process whereby a patient requests a third-party payer to forward its payment for a covered service directly to the physician or other provider of that service; ie, the patient assigns his benefits to that provider.

B

Balance Billing: A process whereby the physician bills a patient for the difference between the physician's charge and the amount of payment already received by the physician from a third-party payer.

Benefit Package: A collection of specific services or benefits that the managed care company is obligated to provide under terms of its contracts with subscriber groups.

Broker: A term generally used to describe one who places insurance business with more than one company and who has no exclusive contract requiring that all his business first be offered to a single company. Unlike the agent, who is considered to represent his company, the broker usually is considered as representing a buyer. Some states, however, make no provisions for the licensing of brokers as such, instead requiring multiple agent-licensing for the broker's placement of business with his various outlets.

C

Capitation: A method of payment for health care services in which the provider accepts a fixed amount of payment per subscriber, per period of time, in return for providing specified services over a specified time period.

Carrier: The party (insurer) to the group contract who agrees to underwrite (carry the risk) and provide certain types of coverage and service.

Case Management: The process by which all health-related matters of a case are managed by a physician or nurse or designated health professional. Physician case managers provide coordination for designated components of the health care, such as appropriate referral to consultants, specialists, hospitals, ancillary providers and services. Case management is intended to ensure continuity of services and accessibility in order to overcome the systems rigidity of many health care systems, fragmented services, misutilization of facilities and resources. It also attempts to match the appropriate intensity of services with the patient's needs over time.

Case Mix: The clinical composition of a hospital's inpatient population among various diagnoses; a factor in determining cost of service and rate setting.

Catastrophic Health Insurance: Insurance beyond basic and major medical insurance for severe and prolonged illness that poses the threat of financial ruin to the family.

Claim Lag: The time interval between incurred date of a claim and its submission to the insurer for payment; also used to mean the time between claim incurral and payment (check or draft issue or redemption).

Claim: A demand by an insured person for the benefits provided by the group contract.

Closed-Panel System: A medical practice in which admission of other doctors is limited by the group and in which members can use only doctors in the group for their medical care. A staff-based HMO is a closed-panel system, while a PPO is an open-panel system.

Coinsurance: That portion of risk borne by the insured as a cash payment. The term differs from "deductible" in that coinsurance can provide first dollar coverage, usually on an 80 percent covered and 20 percent copayment formula.

Community Rating: Determining HMO capitation rates without respect to characteristics or utilization of the subject population. HMOs can vary premium offerings according to benefit packages, but not by health status. Thus, an employed group with characteristics likely to lead to high utilization cannot be charged a higher rate than a group without such characteristics.

Community Rating by Class: A modification of established community rating, whereby individual groups can have different rates depending on the composition by age, sex, marital status, and industry. The changes were included in the 1981 amendments to the federal HMO act affecting qualified plans.

Competitive Medical Plan (CMP): A type of managed care organization created by the 1982 TEFRA legislation to facilitate the enrollment of Medicare beneficiaries into managed care plans. CMPs are organized and financed much like HMOs but are not bound by all the regulatory requirements facing HMOs.

Composite Rate: A uniform premium applicable to all eligibles in a subscriber group regardless of number of claimed dependents. This rate is quite commonplace among labor unions and large employer groups and usually does not require any contribution by the union member or employee.

Concurrent Review: Review of a procedure or hospital admission done by a health care professional other than the one providing the care (usually a nurse).

Contract Size: The number of members per contract.

Contract Mix: The distribution of enrollees according to contracts classified by dependency categories, for example, the number or percentage of singles, doubles, or families. Contract mix is used to determine average contract size.

Conversion Privilege: The right to switch insurance plans on an annual basis regardless of age or physical condition. HMOs must provide an annual renewal period so that their members can remain on a voluntary basis and have the right to convert if they wish. A conversion privilege also refers to the right of an insuree in a group plan to convert to an individual plan if the group plan is canceled.

Coordination of Benefits (COB): A typical insurance provision whereby responsibility for primary payment for medical services is allocated among carriers when a person is covered by more than one employer-sponsored health benefit program. This coordination avoids a person being reimbursed twice for the same medical services.

Copayment: A modest payment made by an HMO enrollee at the time that selected services are rendered. Some HMOs require a $2.00 copayment for each doctor's office call. Some impose a fixed dollar amount for inpatient hospitalization. Copayments are subject to limitation as defined in Subpart A, 110.105 of the Federal HMO Regulations.

Copayment (Copay): An amount of money that the member or insured pays directly to a provider at the time services are rendered.

Cost-Based Reimbursement *(also referred to as retrospective reimbursement):* A method of paying hospitals for actual costs incurred by patients. Those costs must conform to explicit principles defined by third-party payers.

Cost Containment: The control of the overall cost of health care services within the health care delivery system. Costs are contained when the value of the resources committed to an activity is not considered to be excessive.

Cost Effective: A term that refers to the allocation of resources in a manner so as to maximize outcome and minimize cost. There is a point at which more cost will not incrementally improve outcome to the extent of the increased cost. Conversely, less cost will incrementally decrease outcome more than the incremental decreased cost.

Cost Sharing: Responsibility for partial payment by the patient for service rendered. Cost sharing can include:

(a) *Coinsurance,* which is a patient responsibility for payment of a specified *percent* of charges incurred, per day or per unit of service;

(b) *Copayment,* which is a patient responsibility for payment of a specified *dollar amount* per day or per unit of service;

(c) *Deductible,* which is a patient responsibility for payment of a specified amount of incurred expense before third-party coverage can begin.

Cost-Shifting: The phenomenon of passing along costs not paid by one consumer as higher charges to another consumer.

Credentialing: The process of reviewing a practitioner's credentials — ie, training, experience, or demonstrated ability — for the purpose of determining if criteria for clinical privileging are met.

D

Days/1,000/Year: This is a common utilization measurement used in the health care industry that refers to a ratio of the number of days a patient population has for a particular service, most commonly referring to hospital service, per 1,000 members enrolled for a given year. For example, if an HMO had 10,000 members and over a year's period of time they had 3,800 total days in the hospital for those 10,000 members, the ratio then becomes 3,800 for 10,000 patients in a year is equal to 380 hospital days per 1,000 members per year.

Deductibles: Amounts required to be paid by insured as stipulated by contract. For example, all Medicare beneficiaries must satisfy the annual deductible for Part B, Medical Insurance, before entitlement coverage of 80 percent of reasonable medical charges incurred thereafter. The amount paid out-of-pocket is considered a deductible, while the remaining 20 percent of reasonable medical charges is deemed to be the beneficiary's coinsurance level.

Demographics: The statistical characteristics of a defined population (age, sex, income level, race, education, dwellings, employment status, etc) that aid in assessing marketability within that population.

Dependents: Those persons designated in writing by the managed care company enrollee meeting the dependency tests as stipulated in the contract with the subscriber group. Dependency requirements may vary somewhat among contracting subscriber groups of an HMO.

Diagnostic Related Groups (DRGs): A federally mandated program in which hospital procedures are rated in terms of cost, after which a standard flat rate is set per procedure. Medicare claims for those procedures are paid in that amount, regardless of the cost to the hospital.

Differential: The out-of-pocket (or payroll deduction) difference that an eligible individual who opts for insurance coverage may have to pay.

Discounted Fee-for-Service: A financial reimbursement system whereby a provider agrees to provide services on a fee-for-service basis, but with the fees discounted by a certain percentage from the physician's usual charges.

Dual Choice: The opportunity for a consumer within a group to choose from two or more different arrangements for the prepayment of health care, eg, indemnity insurance or an HMO. Section 1310 of the HMO Act and its amendments provide for dual choice.

E

Elective: Usually refers to medical procedures, particularly surgery, not immediately necessary to maintain life or health — procedures that can often be scheduled weeks or months in advance.

Eligibility: Patient status with respect to receiving medical care services as covered benefits.

Enrollee: Anyone enrolled in an HMO and entitled to receive benefits; used synonymously with the term "member."

ERISA: Employee Retirement Income Security Act of 1974, Public Law 93-406. HMOs that contract with firms subject to ERISA compliance can be expected to provide certain annual information to these firms in order to meet federal reporting requirements.

Exclusive Provider Organization (EPO): EPOs are similar to PPOs in their organization and purpose. Unlike PPOs, however, EPOs limit their beneficiaries to participating providers for their health care services. In other words, beneficiaries covered by an EPO are required to receive all of their covered services from providers that participate in the EPO, similar to an HMO. The EPO does not cover services received from other providers. Some EPOs parallel HMOs in that they not only require exclusive use of the EPO provider network, but also use a "gatekeeper" approach to authorize nonprimary care services.

Experience Rating: A method of determining the premium for a health insurance policy based on the average cost of actual or anticipated utilization of care by various groups. Thus, the current premiums take into account age, sex, health status, and so on. Experience rating is not permitted under federal HMO qualification requirements.

F

Federally Qualified HMOs: HMOs that meet certain federally stipulated provisions aimed at protecting consumers — eg, providing a broad range of basic health services, assuring financial solvency, and monitoring the quality of care. HMOs must apply to the federal government for qualification. The process is administered by the Office of Prepaid Health Care of the Health Care Financing Administration (HCFA), Department of Health and Human Services (DHHS).

Fee-for-Service: A system of payment for health care whereby a fee is rendered for each service delivered. Under the fee-for-service system, expenditures increase not only if the fees themselves increase but also if more units of service are charged for or more expensive services are substituted for less expensive ones. This traditional method contrasts with that frequently used in the prepaid sector, where services are covered by a fixed payment made in advance that is independent of the number of services rendered (capitation).

FEHB: Federal Employees Health Benefits program, administered through the US Office of Personnel Management.

First-Dollar Coverage: A policy that, like an HMO, has no deductibles and covers the first dollar of an insuree's expenses.

G

Gatekeeping: The process by which a primary care physician directly provides the primary patient care and coordinates all diagnostic testing and specialty referrals required for a patient's medical care. To receive referrals to specialists and hospitals, the care must be prior-authorized by the "gatekeeper" unless there is an emergency. Gatekeeping is a subset of the functions of the primary physician case manager.

Generic Substitution: Substituting a generic version of a branded off-patent pharmaceutical for the branded product when the latter is prescribed. Some HMOs and Medicaid programs mandate generic substitution. Mandatory generic substitution within the Medicare program is currently being debated in Congress.

Group Contract: An agreement entered into between the managed care company and a subscribing group containing rates, performance covenants, relationships among parties, schedule of benefits, and other conditions. The term is generally limited to a 12-month period and may be renewed after that.

Group or Network HMO: An HMO that contracts with one or more independent group practices to provide services in one or more locations, in which physicians are prepaid on a capitation basis.

Group Practice Model: An HMO model in which the HMO contracts with one or more medical group(s) on a capitation basis for the provision of services. The physicians practice in a common facility and use common staff. Income is pooled and distributed according to an agreed-upon plan.

H

Health Maintenance Organization (HMO): Any organization that, through an organized system of health care, provides or assures the delivery of an agreed-upon set of comprehensive health maintenance and treatment services for an enrolled group of persons under a prepaid fixed sum. Services usually include primary care, emergency care, acute hospital care, extended care, and rehabilitation. To be considered a "Federally Qualified Health Maintenance Organization," the HMO must meet the provisions of the HMO Act, P.L. 93-222, as amended in Title XIII of the Public Health Service Act.

Health Care Financing Administration (HCFA): A division of the Department of Health and Human Services responsible for Medicare and Medicaid.

Health Care Plan: A financial arrangement or organization that provides for the delivery or payment of health care services. Examples include: indemnity health insurance plans, and/or health maintenance organizations (HMOs), employer self-insurance plans, preferred provider organizations (PPOs), and government-sponsored plans (ie, Medicare, Medicaid).

HMO: Health Maintenance Organization.

Hospital Days (per 1,000): A measurement of the utilization of inpatient hospital care per 1,000 population for a specified period of time, usually a year. It is calculated as follows:

Hold Harmless: A clause frequently found in managed care contracts, whereby the HMO and the physician hold each other to be not liable for malpractice or corporate malfeasance if either of the parties is found to be liable. This language does not preclude a managed care company from being sued if one of its physicians is sued. It may also refer to language that prohibits the provider from billing patients in the event a managed care company becomes insolvent. State and federal regulations may require this language.

I

Incentives: As related to medical care delivery, this term refers to economic incentives for providers to motivate efficiency in patient care management.

Incurred But Not Reported Claims (IBNR): Accounting term to represent an appraisal of potential liabilities resulting from the delivery of services that have not been reported as of the time of the report. This is usually caused by delayed submission of claims by hospitals and physicians and other providers. HMOs must keep funds in reserve to cover this liability.

Indemnify: To make good a loss.

Indemnity Insurance: Indemnity insurance typically means coverage offered by insurance companies and Blue Cross plans, whereby individual persons insured are indemnified through reimbursement by the carriers for their medical expenses. Payments may be made to the individual incurring the expense, or, in many cases, directly to providers. The important point is that the indemnity relates only to a specific loss incurred by the insured person after the fact.

Indemnity Carrier: Usually an insurance company or benevolent association that offers selected coverage within a framework of fee schedules, limitations, and exclusions as negotiated with subscriber groups. Insureds are reimbursed after carriers review and process filed claims. Aetna, Connecticut General, and Prudential are examples of indemnity carriers.

Indemnity: A benefit paid by an insurance policy for an insured loss. Often used to refer to benefits paid in cash rather than in terms of services as provided by service-type plans. Also used improperly to denote a benefit payment made without regard to the charges incurred.

Individual Practice Association (IPA): A health maintenance organization delivery model in which the HMO contracts with a physician organization, which, in turn, contracts with individual physicians. The IPA physicians practice in their own offices and continue to see their fee-for-service patients. The HMO reimburses the IPA on a capitated basis; however, the IPA usually reimburses the physicians on a fee-for-service basis. This type of system combines prepayment with the traditional means of delivering health care, ie, physician office/private practice and use of hospitals, nursing homes, and so on.

Intensity Factor: A multiplier or weighting element used in computations to allow for the quantitative influence of a specific variable.

IPA: Individual Practice Association.

L

Length of Stay: The total number of days for which a patient is hospitalized, either totally or in a particular unit or level of care; abbreviated LOS.

Lock-In: An expression referring to an attribute of most HMOs whereby the medical care of a member is not covered by the HMO unless it is rendered by an HMO physician or physician/institution otherwise authorized by the HMO.

Loss Ratio: The ratio between costs incurred for health care services and premiums.

M

Managed Care: A relatively new term coined originally to refer to the prepaid health care sector, (eg, HMOs and CMPs). In general, the term refers to a means of providing health care services within a defined network of health care providers who are given the responsibility to manage and provide quality, cost-effective health care. Increasingly, the term is being used by many analysts to include PPOs and even forms of indemnity insurance coverage that incorporate preadmission certification and other utilization controls.

Managed Care Organization (MCO): A generic term that includes all forms of organizations that provide managed health care services (eg, HMOs, PPOs, CMPs, EPOs, DPOs, PPAs, etc).

Management Information System (MIS): A comprehensive computerized tool that is used for analysis and reporting of important data so that timely, informed decisions can be made.

Market Share: That part of the market potential that a managed care company has captured; usually market share is expressed as a percentage of the market potential.

Medical Director: Physician responsible for bridging health care delivery with management and administration. Major responsibilities include maintaining a provider network, utilization review, and quality assurance.

Medical Group Practice: "Provision of healthcare services by a group of at least three licensed physicians engaged in a formally organized and legally recognized entity; sharing equipment, facilities, common records, and personnel involved in both patient care and business management" is the definition of medical group practice approved by the American Group Practice Association, the American Medical Association, and the Medical Group Management Association.

Medically Necessary: Those covered services required to preserve and maintain the health status of a member or eligible person in accordance with the area standards of medical practice.

Member Month: A unit of volume measurement. A member month is equal to one member enrolled in an HMO for one month, whether or not the member actually receives any services during the period. Two member months are equal to one member enrolled for two months or two members enrolled for one month. Many internal operating statistics for HMOs are expressed in terms of member months.

Member: Anyone enrolled in an HMO and entitled to receive benefits; used synonymously with the term "enrollee."

Multispecialty Group: A group of doctors who represent various medical specialties and who work together in a group practice.

N

Network Model: An organizational form in which the HMO contracts for medical services within a "network" of medical groups. Health Net, a Blue Cross-sponsored HMO serving southern California, is an example of a network model. For federal qualification purposes, such models are designated as IPAs.

Network HMO: See *Group or Network HMO.*

O

Open Enrollment: The time span during which persons in a dual choice health benefits program can select one of the health plans being offered. Also the period referred to in Section 110.107 of the federal qualification regulations during which a federally qualified HMO must make its coverage available without restrictions to individual (nongroup) subscribers who wish to enroll.

Open-Panel HMO: An HMO in which any licensed physician in an area is eligible to join the HMO. An IPA is an example of an open-panel plan.

OPM: Office of Personnel Management, with headquarters in Washington, DC. This agency administers and directs the Federal Employees Health Benefits programs. It is the contracting source for HMOs wishing to become FEHB carriers.

Out-of-Area Benefits: The coverage allowed to HMO members for emergency situations outside of the prescribed geographic area of the HMO.

Out-of-Area-Care: Care received by an HMO's enrollees when they are outside the HMO's geographic territory; services received are usually not prearranged by the HMO.

Out-of-Pocket Payments: Cash payments for services not covered by a third-party payer.

Outcome Audit: A type of patient/medical care evaluation study in which criteria are designed to focus upon desired patient outcome or results of treatment, as distinguished from a process audit in which criteria focus upon the components of appropriate clinical intervention.

Outliers: Patient cases that have either an extremely short or long length of stay or extraordinarily high costs or low costs when compared with most cases classified in the same DRG.

Outpatient: A patient who received medical care services but does not need to be admitted for an overnight stay.

Outside Referral: Referral to a consultant provider not on the managed care company's staff, or not within the group contracting to deliver to the managed care company's professional medical services.

P

P.L. 93-222: Health Maintenance Organization Act of 1973, which created Title XIII of the Public Health Service Act, which established the Federal Health Maintenance Organization program.

P.L. 94-460: The public law that created the 1976 amendments to the Health Maintenance Organization Act of 1973 (Title XIII of the Public Health Service Act, P.L. 93-222). This legislation gave greater flexibility to HMOs in their organization and structure. The amendments also increased federal monies to support HMO development and operation.

Per Diem Rates: A method of payment based on allowable cost per patient day; may encourage longer lengths of stays and increased costs to payers.

Per Diem Cost: Literally, cost per day. Refers, in general, to hospital or other inpatient institutional costs per day or for a day of care. Hospitals occasionally charge for their services on the basis of a per diem rate derived by dividing their total costs by the number of inpatient days of care given. Per diem costs are therefore averages and do not reflect true cost for each patient. Thus, the per diem approach is said to give hospitals an incentive to prolong hospital stays.

Per Member Per Month (PMPM): Refers to the ratio of some service or cost divided into the number of members in a particular group on a monthly basis. For example, if a 10,000 member HMO in one month's time spends $20,000 on cardiovascular surgery, the cost on a PMPM basis would be $20,000 divided by 10,000 equaling $2 per member per month.

Performance Standards: Standards an individual provider is expected to meet, especially with respect to quality of care. The standards may define volume of care delivered per time period. Thus, performance standards for an obstetrician/gynecologist may specify some or all of the following: office hours and office visits per week or month, on-call days, deliveries per year, gynecological operations per year, and so on.

Pre-existing Medical Condition: A physical and/or mental condition that a patient has before applying for insurance coverage. Pre-existing conditions should not affect membership in most HMOs and in some non-HMO group plans.

Pre-existing Conditions Limitation: A restriction on payments on those charges directly resulting from an accident or illness for which the insured received care or treatment within a specified period of time (eg, 3 months) prior to the date he or she became insured.

Preadmission Review: The practice of reviewing claims for inpatient admission before the patient enters the hospital in order to assure that the admission is medically necessary.

Preferred Provider Arrangement (PPA): An arrangement whereby a third-party payer contracts with a group of medical care providers who furnish services at lower than usual fees in return for prompt payment and a certain volume of patients.

Preferred Provider Organization (PPO): PPOs are entities through which employer health benefit plans and health insurance carriers contract to purchase health care services for covered beneficiaries from a selected group of participating providers. Typically, participating providers in PPOs agree to abide by utilization management and other procedures implemented by the PPO, and agree to accept the PPO's reimbursement structure and payment levels. The employer health benefit plans and/or insurance carrier then establish financial incentives in the form of increased benefits for their employees to use the participating preferred hospitals and physicians. In contrast to typical HMO coverage, PPO coverage permits members to use non-PPO providers, although higher levels of coinsurance or deductibles routinely apply to services provided by these nonparticipating providers. PPOs are often formed as a competitive response to HMOs. Some PPOs are now emerging that require providers to share in the financial risk, and others are employing the Gatekeeper concept.

Premium: Used interchangeably with the term "rate"; an expression of the price charged for each class of coverage within a given rate structure. In a broader sense, premium is often used to express the dollar volume contributed by a subscriber group. For example, "That group generated $50,000 in premium last year."

Prepayment: A method of providing the cost of health care services in advance of their use.

Preventive Health Care: Health care that has as its aim the prevention of disease and morbidity before it occurs, and thus concentrates on keeping patients well in addition to healing them when they are sick.

Primary Care: First-level, outpatient, medical services, as opposed to services such as routine surgery for, eg, gallstones (secondary care), or complex medical services and procedures (eg, heart transplants, tertiary care). Primary care sometimes is also defined by the physician specialties involved: Usually family or general practice, pediatrics, obstetrics/gynecology, and internal medicine.

Primary Care Physician (See *Gatekeeping*): A physician who is in some sense a generalist, such as a family practitioner, pediatrician, or general internist. While these physicians deal with the entire person, subspecialist physicians deal only with single body systems — eyes, bones, or skin — or with specific diseases — allergies, diabetes, or heart disease.

Prior Authorization: A method of monitoring/controlling utilization; the evaluation of need and the approval for medical service prior to its being performed, particularly using outside resources.

Provider: Any person or organization involved with providing medical care to consumers. Includes physicians, hospitals, pharmacies, home health agencies, and so on.

Q

Qualification: See *Federally Qualified HMO.*

Quality Assurance: Activities and programs intended to assure the quality of care in a defined medical setting. Such programs must include peer or utilization review components to identify and remedy deficiencies in quality. The program must also have a mechanism for assessing its effectiveness.

Quality of Care: The degree or grade of excellence with respect to medical services received by patients, administered by providers or programs, in terms of technical competence, need, appropriateness, acceptability, humanity, structure, and so on.

R

Reenrollment: In subsequent open enrollment periods, the number of subscribers currently enrolled plus those who elect to join the HMO less those subscribers who leave the HMO, ie, the net number of subscribers who enroll in the HMO.

Reinsurance: A type of protection purchased by some managed care companies from insurance companies specializing in underwriting specific tasks for a stipulated premium. This becomes a cost of doing business for managed care companies. Typical reinsurance risk coverage are: (1) individual stop-loss, (2) aggregate stop-loss, (3) out-of-area, and (4) insolvency protection. As managed care companies grow in membership, they usually reduce their reinsurance coverage (and related direct costs), being in a financial position to assume such risks themselves.

Relative Value Scale (R.V.S.): A guide (not a fee schedule) that attempts to show in a general way by a unit or point designation the relationship between the time, competency, experience, severity, and other factors required to perform one professional service as compared with those required for other professional services, under usual conditions. Such a scale becomes a schedule when dollar conversion factors are applied.

Reserves: Restricted cash investments or highly liquid investments intended to protect the HMO membership against insolvency or bankruptcy. Regulatory agencies may mandate reserve requirements; also, some HMOs establish voluntary reserves by systematically setting aside a small portion of each month's realized revenues.

Risk: The chance or possibility of loss. For example, physicians may be held at risk if hospitalization rates exceed agreed-upon thresholds. The sharing of risk is often employed as a utilization control mechanism within the HMO setting. Risk is also defined in insurance terms as the probability of loss associated with a given population.

Risk Pool: A pool of money that is at risk for being used for defined expenses. Commonly, if the pool of money that is put at risk is not expended by the end of the year, some or all of it is returned to those managing the risk.

Risk Retention: A description of the limitations of financial liability remaining with a major entity to the HMO program. For example, the HMO may accept all risk to guarantee provision of services to its enrolled population. This risk may be limited by arrangements with reinsurers. Also, the fee-for-service/prepaid medical group may take full risk or limit its risk by contractual arrangements with the HMO corporation.

Risk Sharing: Sharing the opportunity for reward or loss. Commonly, physicians and the HMO will share the risk.

S

Same Day Admission: A cost containment procedure that reduces the time a surgical patient spends in the hospital prior to surgery. The preparation for surgery is done as an outpatient.

Self-Insured: Large employers who assume direct responsibility or risk for paying employees' health care without purchasing health insurance. They usually contract with an outside firm to handle claims payment and/or utilization review. Self-insured employers are not required to provide specific benefits and do not pay state insurance tax.

Self-Referrals: Arrangements for care beyond primary care made by the patient rather than the provider. HMOs generally specify to which in-house departments or services a patient may self-refer. For example, patients may be allowed to self-refer to optometry or mental health services. For non-HMO services, patients are not allowed to self-refer if the care is to be paid by the HMO, except in emergencies.

Service Area: The territory within certain boundaries that an HMO designates for providing service to members. Since easy access into the health delivery system is a primary HMO tenet, it is generally believed that a member should not have to drive longer than 30 minutes in order to gain access to the system. Some HMOs establish a mileage radius from their medical delivery sites; some rely on zip codes; others use county boundaries in defining service areas.

Shared Risk: In the context of an HMO, an arrangement in which financial liabilities are apportioned among two or more entities. For example, the HMO and the medical group may each agree to share the risk of excessive hospital cost over budgeted amounts on a 50-50 basis.

Single Contract: Coverage for one person as designated on the enrollment or enrollment change card by the enrollee.

Solvency: A financial condition in which an HMO, a medical group, or another organization is able to pay or retire its debts when due.

Specialty HMO: An HMO organized around a specific medical specialty, such as cancer or cardiac care, that provides prepaid and comprehensive coverage to patients who need it.

Staff Model: The organizational structure of an HMO in which the physicians are salaried employees of the HMO.

Stop-Loss: An arrangement between a managed care company and a reinsurer whereby absorption of prepaid patient expenses are limited, either in terms of overall expenditures and deficit, or by limiting losses on an individual expensive hospital and/or professional services claim.

Subrogation: Seeking, by legal or administrative means, reimbursement from others responsible for certain categories of medical expenses, such as workers' compensation, third-party negligence liability, or no-fault auto medical coverage.

Subscriber: An employer, union, or association that contracts with an HMO for its prepaid health care plan, which is offered to eligible enrollees.

Subspecialist: Someone who is recognized to have expertise in a specialty of medicine or surgery. Within HMOs it usually refers to physicians who are able to receive referrals from primary care physicians.

Supplemental Health Services: The benefits an HMO offers that exceed its basic health service requirements, as defined in Subpart A, 110.101(c) and 110.102 of the Federal HMO Regulations.

T

Tertiary Care: Subspecialty care usually requiring the facilities of a university-affiliated or teaching hospital that has extensive diagnostic and treatment capabilities.

Third-Party Administrator (TPA): Provides services to employers or insurance companies for utilization review, claims payment, and benefit design.

Third-Party Reimbursement: A general term applied to health care benefit payments. It derives from the fact that under normal market transactions, there are only two parties, the consumer and the supplier, but under a benefit plan, a third party (eg, government, an insurance company, an employer, etc) is ultimately responsible to pay the costs of services provided to covered persons.

Third-Party Payer: An organization that acts as a fiscal intermediary between the provider and consumer of care. Examples include: insurance carriers, HMOs, and government as a provider of Medicare and Medicaid.

Three-Tier Rate: A rate structure that sets monthly premiums based on (1) single person coverage; (2) two person coverage; and (3) family coverage.

Title XIX: Commonly refers to the Medicaid program.

Title XVIII: Commonly refers to the Medicare program.

Two-Tier Rate: A rate structure that sets monthly premiums based on (1) single person coverage; and (2) family coverage.

U

Unbundling: Separating a service into its individual components and billing for each component separately. For example, total abdominal hysterectomy billed as five procedures; laporotomy, evaluation under anesthesia, hysterectomy, abdominal exploration, and oophorectomy. Also referred to as a trend in insurance benefits contracting wherein the purchaser unbundles or contracts separately for specific services (eg, mental health, dental care, etc).

Underwriting: The process of selecting, classifying, evaluating, and assuming risks according to their insurability.

Usual, Customary and Reasonable (UCR): Health insurance plans that pay a physician's full charge if it does not exceed his usual charge, does not exceed the amount customarily charged for the service by other physicians in the area, or is otherwise reasonable.

Utilization Management (Utilization Review, Utilization Control): Systematic means for reviewing and controlling patients' use of medical care services, and providers' use of medical care resources. Usually involves data collection, review and/or authorization, especially for services such as specialist referrals and emergency room use, and particularly costly services such as hospitalization.

Utilization Review: System of review conducted by professional personnel of the appropriateness, quality of, and need for health care services rendered to patients.

Utilization: The patterns of rates of use of a service or type of service within a specified time. Utilization is generally expressed in rates per unit of population-at-risk for a given period, eg, the number of admissions to a hospital per 1,000 persons enrolled in an HMO per year.

V

Value: A function of both the cost and quality of a product or service.

Voluntary Enrollment: The nature of how patients come to be HMO members — they consciously and explicitly choose to enroll. Further, HMO membership is almost always offered as one of at least two health coverage options, whereas insurance is sometimes the only offered option.

W

Withhold: The portion of the monthly capitation payment to physicians withheld by an HMO until the end of the year or other time period to create an incentive for efficient care. The withhold is "at risk." If the physician (or group of physicians) exceeds utilization norms, he does not receive it. It serves as a financial incentive for lower utilization. The withhold can cover all services or be specific to hospital care, laboratory usage, or specialty referrals.

Sources

American Medical Association, "Glossary of Terms Related to Physician Payment," 1984.

Discursive Dictionary of Health Care, US Government Printing Office, 1976.

Harris, John M., *The Role of the Medical Director in the Fee-for-Service/ Prepaid Medical Group.* Denver, CO: Center for Research in Ambulatory Health Care Administration, 1983.

Marketing Seminar for Health Maintenance Organizations, course materials, presented by Office of Health Maintenance Organizations, Department of Health, Education, and Welfare. Adapted from Jurgovan and Blair, Inc. January 1980.

Minnesota Medical Association, "Health Care Competition Paper," 1983.

National Health Lawyers Association, "1988 Managed Care: Risk, Challenge, and Opportunity, A Managed Care Primer: An Overview of the Organization, Operation, and Financing of HMO and PPO Plans."

Neal, Patricia A., *Management Information Systems for the Fee-for-Service/ Prepaid Medical Group.* Denver, CO: Center for Research in Ambulatory Health Care Administration, 1983, reprinted 1986.

Office of Health Maintenance Organizations, Public Health Service, Department of Health and Human Services, *HMO Governing Board Handbook,* April 1981.

Society of Teachers of Family Medicine, "Managed Health Care: A Teaching Syllabus," prepared by the Task Force on Managed Health Care. Kansas City, MO: May 1990.

Sutton, Harry L. and Allen J. Sorbo, *Actuarial Issues in the Fee-for-Service/ Prepaid Medical Group.* Denver, CO: Center for Research in Ambulatory Health Care Administration, 1983, reprinted 1986.

About the Author

David Vogel is a graduate of the Universities of Wisconsin and Colorado who holds undergraduate and graduate degrees in industrial psychology, health administration, and health planning. His experience in the health care field includes almost 25 years in managed care as a chief executive and a consultant. He has provided consultative services regarding managed care to more than 400 health care organizations in 46 states.

The author has also facilitated workshops, seminars, and retreats for physicians and other providers throughout the country on the subject of how to survive and thrive in the managed care arena. He is a frequent speaker on managed care at regional and national meetings, and is recognized as one of the nation's leading experts on the subject.

e

9/